Sexual Health and Wellbeing: A Holistic Handbook for Women's Intimacy, Fulfillment and Authentic Expression

PUBLISHED BY Golden Folio Editions

© Copyright 2024 - All rights reserved.

Table of contents

Introduction

"Sexuality is one of the most profound ways we connect—to ourselves, to others, and to life itself."

From the first flush of desire to the gentle afterglow of shared vulnerability, our sexual selves inform every facet of our being. Yet too often, conversations about women's sexual health are relegated to the realm of dysfunction or framed exclusively as erotic spectacle. This handbook seeks to reclaim sexuality in its fullest dimensions—physical, emotional, social, and spiritual—positioning it not as a narrow performance or fetishized fantasy, but as an essential thread in the fabric of holistic wellbeing. Here, you will find an invitation to explore your unique landscape of pleasure, to cultivate informed consent and authentic connection, and to integrate creative rituals that honor your body's wisdom throughout every stage of life.

Defining Holistic Sexual Health

At its heart, "holistic sexual health" is the seamless integration of four interwoven dimensions:

1. **Physical**: Understanding the anatomy of arousal, the rhythms of our hormones, and the neurobiological pathways that give rise to sensation.
2. **Emotional**: Nurturing the tender terrain of vulnerability, attachment, and self-worth that shapes our capacity to feel seen, safe, and satisfied.
3. **Social**: Cultivating clear communication, enthusiastic consent, and ethical negotiation with partners, communities, and ourselves.
4. **Spiritual**: Honoring sexuality as a sacred expression of life force, a conduit for creativity, ritual, and transcendent connection.

By contrast, this guide does not delve into fetish-specific practices or purely erotic scripts. While pleasure and sensuality are central, our focus remains on education, empowerment, and lifelong wellbeing. You will learn evidence-based insights— from the latest neuroendocrine research to proven somatic therapies—alongside creative exercises that invite curiosity, play, and self-discovery. Whether you are seeking greater intimacy with a partner, deeper self-knowledge in solo practice, or a richer intersection between sexuality and spirituality, this book will serve as your compass.

Who This Guide Is For—and How to Use It

This handbook is crafted for adult women (18 years and older) who are ready to claim agency over their sexual lives. If you have ever felt unseen by mainstream sexual health resources, intimidated by medicalized language, or curious about broadening your repertoire of intimate skills, you are in the right place. We intentionally flag this as "Adult, but not erotic" material: while frank discussions of anatomy, pleasure, and consensual practices are woven throughout, our approach is deeply respectful, body-positive, and devoid of gratuitous titillation. You will never find sensationalized descriptions here—only clear, compassionate guidance designed to empower you to make informed choices and to celebrate your sexuality as an integral part of overall health.

Throughout these pages, the tone will be that of an encouraging mentor: knowledgeable yet never condescending, clinical when necessary but always accessible, scientific yet infused with warmth. You are invited to move at your own pace, to pause and reflect, and to adapt practices to your individual preferences and cultural context. Exercises are presented as optional experiments rather than mandates—your body, your boundaries, your journey.

The Journey Ahead: From Self-Awareness to Authentic Expression

This book is structured as a progressive voyage, beginning at the center of your own experience and radiating outward toward connection with others and engagement with wider communities. Briefly, here is how you will travel:

- **Part I: Embodied Self**

  We begin by illuminating the mind-body nexus: the neurobiology of pleasure, somatic awareness techniques, and the role of stress regulation in sustaining desire. You will gain tools to tune into subtle bodily signals, to modulate your nervous system, and to honor the intelligence encoded in every nerve ending.

- **Part II: Mapping Your Pleasure Blueprint**

  Next, you will chart a personalized pleasure map, uncovering the unique constellation of sensations, contexts, and emotional states that unlock your deepest arousal. Through guided journaling, sensory experiments, and cultural deconstruction, you will dismantle old narratives and build a pleasure profile tailored to your evolving tastes.

- **Part III: Communication, Consent & Negotiation**

  With self-knowledge as your foundation, you will learn to articulate desires, negotiate boundaries, and co-create consensual experiences. From verbal consent frameworks to nonverbal attunement, digital tools for tracking boundaries to embodied check-ins, you will discover how clarity and compassion can transform sexual interactions.

- **Part IV: Emotional Intimacy & Attachment Styles**

  Here we explore the emotional substratum of desire: attachment patterns formed in childhood that continue to shape adult sexuality. You will engage in vulnerability rituals, gratitude ceremonies, and trauma-healing protocols that foster secure attachment and deepen relational trust.

- **Part V: Body Positivity & Self-Image**

  Recognizing that body dissatisfaction undermines sexual confidence for many women, we dedicate a section to media literacy, mirror work, and playful movement practices that celebrate every curve, line, and gesture of embodied self-love.

- **Part VI: Hormonal Health Across the Lifespan**

  Desire ebbs and flows in tandem with hormonal cycles— from the first period to the second bloom of menopause. You will learn to observe cyclical rhythms, anticipate shifting patterns of libido, and make informed decisions about contraception, hormone replacement, and cycle syncing.

- **Part VII: Holistic Practices for Sexual Wellbeing**

  In this section, integrative modalities take center stage: pelvic-floor yoga, dance flows, breathwork, meditation, nutritional support, and somatic therapies that together nurture a resilient, responsive sexual system.

- **Part VIII: Integrating Sexuality with Overall Wellness**

Sexual health does not exist in isolation. We examine how fitness, sleep hygiene, mental health, and social support synergize with your intimate life, offering practical strategies to weave sexuality seamlessly into your daily routines.

- **Part IX: Sexual Empowerment & Agency**

  Agency is the cornerstone of fulfilling sex: you will confront shame and guilt, build confidence through deliberate practice, and learn to advocate for yourself and others in personal relationships and on a collective level.

- **Part X: Authentic Expression & Creative Rituals**

  Finally, the book culminates in a celebration of creativity, ritual, and future-facing technology. You will discover how erotic art, vision-boarding, moon-cycle ceremonies, and emerging VR or AI tools can invigorate your sexual expression and expand the boundaries of possibility.

Each chapter combines concise theoretical overviews, step-by-step protocols, reflective prompts, and curated resources— delivered in a friendly, conversational voice that respects your intelligence and autonomy. Throughout, you will find case vignettes illustrating real women's journeys, evidence-based sidebars highlighting key research findings, and "Try This" callouts to guide your personal experiments.

A Note on Language and Inclusivity

While this handbook centers women's experiences, we honor the fullness of gender diversity: the trans and nonbinary community often face barriers to receiving comprehensive sexual health education, and many of the practices herein may be adapted to support a wide spectrum of bodies and identities. We use the term "women" to reference those who identify as such, but we encourage all readers to interpret and modify suggestions in accordance with their own gender identity and lived realities.

You will also encounter inclusive language around relationships, recognizing that intimacy may unfold within monogamous partnerships, polyamorous networks, solo exploration, or relational configurations that defy categorization. Wherever possible, we present examples across these contexts and invite you to situate each practice within your own relational map.

Why Holistic Sexual Health Matters

A growing body of research underscores what many women have felt intuitively: when sexual health is nurtured holistically, the benefits ripple through every aspect of life. Enhanced self-esteem, deeper emotional bonds, reduced stress, improved cardiovascular health, greater creative vitality, and even spiritual awakening have all been linked to a vibrant sexual life. Conversely, sexual neglect or unresolved trauma can impair mental health, strain relationships, and diminish overall wellbeing.

This handbook is grounded in the conviction that sexuality, properly understood and practiced, is not a luxury or a mere source of pleasure—it is an essential human need, on par with nourishment, sleep, and meaningful connection. By weaving together cutting-edge science, timeless wisdom traditions, and radical body-affirming practices, we aim to equip you with a sustainable framework for sexual flourishing that will serve you for a lifetime.

Your Invitation

As you turn these pages, I invite you to approach each chapter with an open mind and a spirit of experimentation. There is no "one right way" to experience pleasure or intimacy; the path you carve will be as unique as your fingerprints. Some exercises may click immediately, others may require repeated visits or creative adaptation. You might discover new desires you never anticipated—and that, too, is a triumph of self-awareness.

Keep a dedicated journal or digital record as you journey through this handbook. Note sensations, shifts in mood, breakthroughs, and obstacles. Share insights with trusted friends, partners, or a supportive community, if you choose. Above all, practice self-compassion: every step toward deeper embodiment and authentic expression is valuable, regardless of outcome.

Looking Ahead

In the chapters that follow, you will not only learn about your body's hormones, neural circuits, and musculoskeletal dynamics—you will also cultivate the emotional intelligence, communicative clarity, and creative courage to bring those insights into your daily life. Whether you embark solo or with a partner, equipped with curiosity and respect, you will soon find that sexual wellbeing is not a static achievement but an ever-evolving tapestry woven from each experience of pleasure, connection, and growth.

May this handbook serve as your guide, your companion, and your catalyst for profound transformation. Welcome to a journey of self-discovery that honors your body, celebrates your desires, and connects you more deeply to the life force pulsing within and around you.

Chapter 1: Embodied Self – The Mind-Body Connection

"Your brain is the most powerful sexual organ"—over 50% of sexual response originates in the neural pathways.

Sexual experience unfolds not just in the genitals or erogenous zones but through a cascade of signals that flow between body and brain. Understanding this intricate dialogue helps demystify arousal, attachment, and pleasure. In this chapter, we launch our journey at the neural interface, exploring how neurochemicals guide desire, how women's brains uniquely process pleasure, and how the health of our gut influences mood and libido.

1.1 Neurobiology of Pleasure

Pleasure is both universal and deeply personal. Whether it arises in response to a gentle caress, an intimate embrace, or solitary self-exploration, the sensations we label "pleasurable" are orchestrated by chemical messengers, specialized brain regions, and even the trillions of microbes that inhabit our digestive tract. By mapping these systems, we gain tools to cultivate wellbeing: we learn why stress blocks desire, how bonding hormones deepen connection, and how a balanced microbiome can support a vibrant sex drive.

Mapping Dopamine, Oxytocin, and Endorphin Circuits

At the heart of every pleasurable sensation lies a trio of neurochemicals:

- **Dopamine**: Often called the "motivation molecule," dopamine surges when we anticipate reward. In sexual contexts, it sharpens focus and drives exploration. When you set an intention to connect—mentally or physically—dopamine pathways light up, heightening sensitivity to touch, scent, and sight. This neurotransmitter also reinforces learning: positive sexual experiences strengthen the neural circuits that guide us back to pleasure.
- **Oxytocin**: Dubbed the "bonding hormone," oxytocin floods the bloodstream during intimate contact—skin-to-skin warmth, eye gazing, and especially orgasm. It promotes feelings of safety and trust by dampening the activity of the amygdala, the brain's fear center. After release, oxytocin fosters emotional closeness, making partners feel more attuned and affectionate. In solo practice, self-administered touch can likewise prompt oxytocin release, reinforcing a sense of self-compassion and body acceptance.
- **Endorphins**: These natural opioids act as the body's painkillers and mood elevators. They are particularly active during sustained or rhythmic stimulation—think prolonged eye contact, synchronized breathing, or steady pelvic movements. Endorphins soothe tension in muscles and promote a calm euphoria, often referred to as the "afterglow."

These three neurochemicals do not act in isolation. Rather, they interact in feedback loops: dopamine primes the system by building anticipation; oxytocin takes the baton, creating intimate connection; and endorphins carry us over the finish line into contentment and relaxation. This sequence explains why building sexual tension—through flirting, teasing, or slow, deliberate touch—can intensify the eventual release and deepen the sense of closeness that follows.

Gender-Specific Neural Activation Patterns

Functional magnetic resonance imaging (fMRI) has revealed that women's brains often engage multiple regions simultaneously when processing sexual stimuli:

- **Reward Centers**: The nucleus accumbens and ventral tegmental area, central to the dopamine pathway, show robust activation. In women, these regions may be more sensitive to contextual cues—emotional safety, relationship quality, and psychological comfort—than in men.
- **Emotional and Memory Hubs**: Areas such as the hippocampus (involved in memory consolidation) and the anterior cingulate cortex (integrating emotion and decision-making) are more frequently recruited. This suggests that for many women, pleasure is woven together with emotional context and past experiences. A supportive environment, positive self-image, and a trusting partner can literally amplify neural response.
- **Sensory and Motor Areas**: The somatosensory cortex (which processes touch and bodily sensations) and the supplementary motor area (involved in planning movement) often co-activate, reflecting the intricate interplay between mind and body. This neural coupling may underlie why activities that combine movement, such as dance or focused breathwork, can enhance sexual readiness and responsiveness.

Importantly, these patterns exhibit considerable individual variation. Hormonal status, life stage (e.g., menstrual phase, pregnancy, menopause), and personal history (including trauma or chronic stress) all modulate neural responsiveness. For instance, during the pre-ovulatory window—when estrogen peaks—women often report heightened arousal and a slight shift in brain activation toward the reward circuitry. Conversely, phases characterized by higher progesterone may lean the system toward relaxation and bonding, with oxytocin pathways taking prominence.

By recognizing that women's neural processing of pleasure is dynamic and context-dependent, we affirm that there is no "right" speed or style. Some may find deep emotional resonance amplifies arousal; others may thrive on novel sensory exploration. Both paths engage the brain's pleasure machinery— each through its own route.

The Gut-Brain Axis and Sexuality

Emerging research underscores a surprising player in our sexual wellbeing: the gut microbiome. The millions of bacteria, viruses, and fungi residing in our intestines communicate bidirectionally with the brain via the vagus nerve, immune signals, and microbial metabolites. Here's how gut health influences libido and mood regulation:

1. **Neurotransmitter Production**
   - Certain gut bacteria synthesize precursors to serotonin, the "feel-good" neurotransmitter. While most serotonin acts in the digestive tract to regulate motility, a fraction crosses the blood-brain barrier or influences peripheral receptors that modulate mood and anxiety—key factors in

sexual desire. Low serotonin levels are strongly linked to depressive symptoms, which often correlate with diminished libido.

2. **Inflammation and Immune Signaling**
   o An imbalanced microbiome ("dysbiosis") can trigger low-grade inflammation. Chronic inflammation elevates cytokines that cross into the brain and may dampen dopamine signaling, reducing motivation and pleasure sensitivity. By contrast, a diverse gut flora supports regulatory immune pathways that protect neural health and preserve a robust reward response.

3. **Hormonal Metabolism**
   o The gut participates in the enterohepatic circulation of sex hormones. Certain bacterial species produce enzymes that influence estrogen reactivation in the intestines, thereby affecting systemic levels. Dysbiosis can impair this recycling, potentially leading to estrogen dominance or deficiency—both of which can disrupt sexual function, vaginal health, and mood stability.

4. **Stress Responsivity**
   o The microbiome shapes the body's reactivity to stress by modulating the hypothalamic-pituitary-adrenal (HPA) axis. A resilient gut ecosystem can buffer cortisol release, preventing the stress-induced suppression of libido. Practices that support microbial diversity—such as a fiber-rich diet, fermented foods, and moderate exercise—thus become indirect allies in maintaining sexual desire under pressure.

By tending the gut as part of a holistic self-care regimen, women can support both mental wellbeing and sexual vitality. Simple interventions—probiotic-rich yogurt, prebiotic foods like garlic and onions, and mindful eating to encourage parasympathetic activation—lay the groundwork for a thriving microbiome. Over time, improvements in digestion, sleep, and mood often translate into a rekindled interest in intimacy.

Putting It into Practice

Understanding these neurobiological foundations empowers you to craft daily rituals that feed your pleasure pathways:

1. **Anticipation Rituals (Dopamine Boost)**
   o Schedule small moments of anticipation: send a flirtatious text to your partner, linger over an alluring scent, or envision a sensual scene in a journal. These micro-doses of excitement prime dopamine circuits, making later touch feel more intense.
2. **Connection Rituals (Oxytocin Activation)**
   o Incorporate non-sexual skin-to-skin contact into your routine: partner massages, cuddling with a pet, or gentle self-massage with lubricating oils. Even brief moments of warmth and pressure on the chest or belly can encourage oxytocin release and deepen your capacity for attachment.
3. **Flow Rituals (Endorphin Release)**
   o Engage in rhythmic movement practices—yoga flows that emphasize pelvic mobility, synchronized partner breathing sessions, or slow, deliberate dance. Aim for at least 10 minutes of continuous, rhythmic activity to tap endorphin circuits that calm the nervous system.
4. **Brain-Body Synchrony (Mindful Awareness)**

- Cultivate interoceptive attention through guided body scans or mindful breathing. By learning to notice subtle changes—heart rate shifts, muscle tension, or temperature differences—you strengthen the pathways that link sensory input to emotional and cognitive responses.

5. **Gut-Friendly Habits**
   - Build microbial diversity with fermented foods (sauerkraut, kefir), prebiotic-rich fibers (bananas, asparagus), and polyphenol sources (berries, dark chocolate). Pair meals with relaxation techniques—deep breathing or brief meditation—to favor parasympathetic digestion and optimize nutrient absorption.

As you integrate these insights and practices, remember that neurobiology is not destiny. Your experience of pleasure is as much shaped by relationships, cultural narratives, and personal history as by chemical messengers. Yet by illuminating the internal mechanisms at work, we gain powerful levers to enhance wellbeing: we choose foods that feed our microbiome, rituals that quiet stress, and movements that awaken endorphins. In the next section, we turn outward from the microscopic to the somatic, exploring how mindful touch, myofascial release, and progressive relaxation further prime the body for receptive, joyful intimacy.

1.2 Somatic Awareness Practices

Developing a refined awareness of the body's internal landscape—known as interoception—is the cornerstone of somatic practice. When we slow down long enough to notice subtle shifts in tension, temperature, or trembling, we awaken an inner dialogue that can profoundly deepen our capacity for pleasure and safety. One of the most accessible gateways to this dialog is the body scan. In its simplest form, a body scan invites you to lie or sit in a comfortable position and direct your attention, in turn, to different regions of the anatomy: perhaps beginning at the crown of the head, tracing down through the jaw, neck, shoulders, and spine, and arriving finally at the feet. As you move your focus, allow yourself to notice sensations without judgment—warmth under your shoulder blades, an echo of tension behind the knees, the gentle ebb and flow of breath in the belly. Over time, practicing this technique for ten minutes a day cultivates a map of habitual holding patterns: the habitual tightening of the jaw under stress, the unexamined grip of tension around the ribcage, the way the pelvis may tilt forward or clench closed. By simply observing these patterns, we begin to create space for choice rather than default reactivity.

Once the foundational skill of scanning has taken root, the practice of mindful touch offers a bridge between cognitive awareness and embodied sensation. Mindful touch is neither a performance nor a goal-oriented act; rather, it is an exploratory conversation with the body. You might begin by placing one hand lightly over your heart, noticing the subtlest rhythm of your heartbeat, the warmth of your palm against your chest, and any emotional responses that arise. Then, allow your hand to drift to your abdomen, the sinewy curve of your waist, the front of your thighs. At each resting point, pause and breathe, listening for undercurrents of tension or relaxation. The intention is not to arouse or to seek pleasure per se, but to cultivate a language of sensation so that, when you do engage in intimate touch—whether with a partner or in self-exploration—you are fluent in the body's nuanced vocabulary. Over weeks of practice, many women report a greater ability to detect the first flickers of arousal or relaxation, to notice when the pelvis wishes to soften or to tilt, or to discern the precise quality of pressure or movement that feels nourishing rather than overwhelming.

While mindful touch and body scanning are self-guided and introspective, hands-on therapies such as Rolfing and myofascial release offer targeted interventions to release tension stored deep in the connective tissues. The pelvic floor in particular, a hammock of muscles and fascia at the base of the torso, can become chronically tight due to stress, poor posture, or past injuries. Rolfing, a form of structural integration, employs sustained pressure and movement to reorganize the body's tissues in relation to gravity. During a session, a practitioner will apply firm, yet sensitive, pressure along the fascial lines that envelop the pelvis, guiding the fascia to lengthen and soften. Many women describe a potent sense of unblocking, as though an old knot of tension has gently unwound, creating newly available space and ease of movement.

Myofascial release, by contrast, can be self-administered using tools such as soft balls, foam rollers, or specialized pelvic wands. In this practice, the focus is on locating areas of tightness—often a tender or "trigger" point—and maintaining steady, unhurried pressure while breathing deeply. The sensation may range from mild discomfort to a profound "ah" of release, but the essential principle is patience: fascia responds not to force but to time. Fifteen to twenty seconds of sustained, gentle pressure can prompt the tissue fibers to reorganize, restoring elasticity and reducing the reflexive guarding that inhibits pelvic mobility. As the pelvic floor resumes a balanced tone—neither excessively tight nor lax—many women notice greater comfort in daily movements, an enhanced sense of grounding, and a more responsive somatic foundation for intimate connection.

These somatic interventions reach their full potential when integrated into a broader framework of relaxation. Progressive muscle relaxation (PMR), originally developed to reduce anxiety, can be adapted specifically to prime the nervous system for sexual readiness. In PMR, the practitioner or the individual systematically tenses and then releases muscle groups, often beginning with the feet and ascending to the head or vice versa. To tailor this for embodied self-work, one might begin by curling the toes tightly, holding for a count of five, then releasing with a sigh and noticing the wave of softness that follows. Next, attention shifts to the calves, thighs, glutes, lower back, and so on, always pairing the act of tension with mindful release. What differentiates a sexuality-focused adaptation of PMR is the pacing and the locus of attention: rather than rushing through twelve muscle groups in ten minutes, allow yourself to linger in areas where tension feels most pronounced—perhaps the pelvic floor, the inner thighs, or the lower abdomen. Permit each release to be accompanied by slow, belly-centered breathing, letting each exhale carry away residual tension. Over time, this practice tunes the autonomic nervous system to move smoothly out of fight-or-flight arousal into a state of receptive calm—the parasympathetic mode that underlies easeful pleasure.

The synergistic effect of these somatic practices cannot be overstated. Body scanning builds interoceptive literacy; mindful touch translates awareness into gentle exploration; Rolfing and myofascial release restore structural freedom; and progressive muscle relaxation reprograms the nervous system's baseline. Collectively, they forge a resilient platform from which desire can arise unimpeded by chronic tension or stress. With each moment of practiced presence, the body learns to cradle sensation rather than resist it—and it is in that cradle of safety and curiosity that truly embodied intimacy can flourish.

1.3 Stress, Autonomic Regulation & Libido

In our fast-paced world, stress has become a ubiquitous companion—yet its subtle, chronic presence can undermine sexual desire in ways that often go unrecognized. The autonomic nervous system, a network of neural circuits governing involuntary functions, operates chiefly through two complementary branches: the sympathetic ("fight, flight, or freeze") and the parasympathetic ("rest and digest" or "tend and befriend"). Polyvagal theory, pioneered by Dr. Stephen Porges, adds nuance by distinguishing between a dorsal vagal complex that can induce shutdown states and a ventral vagal complex that supports social engagement and co-regulation. For sexual wellbeing, activating the ventral vagal pathway is essential, since this branch fosters feelings of safety, connection, and openness to sensation.

Practically speaking, vagal stimulation need not involve esoteric rituals. Simple practices—such as gentle humming, chanting, or prolonged exhalations—can engage the vagus nerve, the cranial highway connecting the brainstem to the heart, lungs, and gut. Even the act of slow, diaphragmatic breathing, with an intentional pause at the bottom of the exhale, can modulate vagal tone and shift the body away from threat-response patterns. As the vagus nerve gently coaxes the heart rate downward and invites the digestive organs to resume normal function, women often report a palpable easing in pelvic tension and a more vivid sense of bodily presence. In partner settings, mutual support of these practices—sitting back-to-back in synchronized breathing, for instance—can further amplify co-regulation, reminding both individuals that they are, in Porges's words, "safe enough to feel."

Yet chronic stress is not merely a psychological state; it orchestrates biochemical cascades that impinge directly on sexual hormones. Cortisol, the body's principal stress hormone, is indispensable in short bursts—mobilizing energy, sharpening focus, and modulating inflammation. However, when cortisol remains elevated day after day, it exerts a suppressive effect on the hypothalamic-pituitary-gonadal axis, the hormonal symphony controlling estrogen, progesterone, and testosterone production. For women, this suppression can mean irregular menstrual cycles, diminished vaginal lubrication, and a muted drive for intimacy. Moreover, cortisol's sway over blood sugar regulation and immune function can exacerbate mood swings, fatigue, and body-image concerns, creating a downward spiral that further dampens desire.

To mitigate these effects, a multi-pronged approach is essential. Nutritional strategies focus on stabilizing blood sugar—eating balanced meals rich in fiber, protein, and healthy fats to prevent cortisol spikes triggered by hypoglycemia. Incorporating adaptogenic herbs such as ashwagandha or rhodiola can offer gentle support to the adrenal system, smoothing cortisol fluctuations without the side effects of potent stimulants. From a lifestyle perspective, carving out daily periods of restorative activity—be it a midday walk unaccompanied by screens, a ten-minute meditation practice, or an evening ritual of reading by candlelight—signals to the body that not all moments are crises. By reinforcing the message that relaxation is permitted, we gradually recalibrate the HPA axis toward greater equilibrium, allowing reproductive hormones to resume their natural cadence.

Even with these behavioral and nutritional supports in place, it can be challenging to gauge progress in the abstract realm of "stress reduction." Heart rate variability (HRV) biofeedback offers an objective window into autonomic regulation. HRV measures the variation in time between successive heartbeats—a higher variability indicates greater parasympathetic activity and a more flexible, adaptive nervous system. Today's wearable devices and smartphone apps can track HRV trends, providing real-time feedback on how quickly the body recovers after a stressful event or how deeply it settles into rest. Protocols for improving HRV often begin with coherence breathing, a paced rhythm of about six breaths per minute, which has been shown to maximize vagal engagement. As HRV readings rise over weeks of practice, many women observe parallel shifts in their subjective experience: less pelvic discomfort before intimacy, quicker recovery from performance anxiety, and a more spontaneous emergence of desire.

Integrating HRV biofeedback into a comprehensive stress-management plan transforms abstract goals into tangible milestones. Rather than relying on willpower alone to "relax," you work in partnership with your physiology, gradually shaping neural pathways that favor openness over contraction. In a culture that prizes productivity above all, HRV data can serve as a gentle reminder that your nervous system—forged across millennia to respond to real threats—is ready to embrace pleasure and connection when given the chance.

Taken together, the principles of polyvagal theory, cortisol management, and HRV training illuminate a path through the thicket of stress toward renewed libido and embodied ease. By intentionally engaging the ventral vagal system, bolstering hormonal balance through diet and lifestyle, and tracking progress with biofeedback tools, we reclaim the autonomic terrain as a fertile ground for sexual flourishing rather than a battleground of chronic arousal. In the next chapter, we will build upon this regulated foundation by mapping personalized pleasure blueprints—structures that translate newfound physiological freedom into creative, context-specific pathways for joy and intimacy.

Chapter 2: Mapping Your Pleasure Blueprint

"Only 15% of women report fully understanding what brings them consistent pleasure—yet personalized 'pleasure maps' can boost orgasm frequency by 40%."

To navigate toward more reliable, fulfilling experiences, it helps to view pleasure not as a vague ideal but as a territory that can be charted. Just as a landscape survey reveals hidden valleys and high points, a pleasure map illuminates the body's unique contours of sensitivity, the contexts that enliven desire, and the emotional currents that accompany arousal. In this chapter, we guide you through the process of creating your own personalized pleasure map—a dynamic tool that evolves with you over time. By combining structured reflection, creative visualization, and systematic experimentation, you will uncover patterns and preferences that often lie buried beneath cultural scripts or scattered memories.

2.1 Creating a Personal Pleasure Map

The first step in constructing a pleasure map is to gather data on the experiences that have felt most enlivening. Rather than relying on general impressions ("I like kissing," "I enjoy warmth"), we will approach memory with precision. You may begin by opening a journal and writing in response to prompts that encourage you to recall concrete moments when your body felt heightened, soft, or otherwise awakened. For instance, you might describe a sensation you experienced during a summer evening breeze brushing across your skin, noting precisely which part of your torso felt electric, how your breathing shifted, what thoughts or memories flickered in your mind, and which emotions—joy, curiosity, longing—surfaced. In another reflection, you could recall a time when you felt enlivened by a certain fragrance or sound: perhaps the rich aroma of brewing coffee, the distant rhythm of rain on a windowpane, or the resonance of a particular piece of music. In each description, attend not only to what you sensed in the body but also to the context—the environment, your posture, your emotional state, and even the social setting if others were present. Over a series of such journal entries, patterns begin to emerge: certain textures, temperatures, or rhythms that consistently spark tingles of pleasure, shifts in mood, or gentle pulses of anticipation.

While freewriting allows for rich, nuanced recollections, structure can help capture data in a form that is easier to compare over time. On the page beside your narrative reflections, create a simple table with columns for "Date," "Memory or Experiment," "Region of Sensation," "Intensity (1–10)," and "Emotional Quality." Although the map's ultimate form will be visual rather than tabular, this preliminary framework provides a quick-reference record. As you fill in each row, you begin to quantify your experience: Was the pleasure fleeting or lingering? Did it arise in the lower back, along the collarbone, at the nape of the neck? Did it coincide with feelings of safety, excitement, nostalgia, or playful curiosity? Over time, these entries may reveal surprising trends: perhaps the inner wrists respond more strongly to gentle, circular movement than the fingertips, or the softness of cotton against the skin triggers more resonance than silk. Writing down these specifics transforms abstract impressions into actionable insights.

Once you have gathered several weeks of journal entries and tabled observations, the next phase is to translate this data into a visual form. On a large sheet of paper, or in a digital drawing program, sketch an outline of the human body in a neutral stance—either front-facing or in multiple views. You might label the outline simply "Pleasure Blueprint" and date the initial draft. Using colored pencils or digital brushes, mark the areas where you recorded the highest intensity scores. Warm hues, like reds and oranges, can denote regions of particularly intense response; cooler tones, such as blues or greens, can indicate areas of more subtle sensitivity. Don't shy away from layering colors: a region that responded variably—sometimes intense, sometimes mild—can be shaded in overlapping tones, conveying the fluidity of experience. Around the edges of the outline, annotate any contextual notes: a small star by the region where you felt a warm knot of pleasure while watching a sunset, or a wavy line by the ankles recalling the tickle of water lapping at your skin.

If you find that certain sensations do not map neatly to static body zones—perhaps you experience pleasurable waves that sweep diagonally across your torso—you can draw arrows or flow lines to represent the direction and movement of sensation. Energy-flow diagrams, borrowed from somatic traditions, can deepen your understanding of how pleasure travels. For example, you might notice that a gentle massage of the abdomen sends ripples of warmth upward toward the chest; by drawing an upward arrow, you capture that dynamic. Similarly, a grounding pressure at the soles of your feet might radiate upward through the legs; a set of vertical lines can communicate that rising energy. The goal is to create a living, breathing blueprint that speaks to both location and movement.

With an initial map sketched out, the process moves into its experiment-and-refine phase. Over a six-week cycle, you will design short, focused sessions—each lasting no more than fifteen or twenty minutes—during which you actively explore specific regions or modalities. One week might be devoted to temperature contrasts: you gently apply a cool cloth to one marked zone and a warmed pack or your own warmed hands to another, observing how intensity ratings shift in your journal table. Another week might invite you to experiment with textures: soft fur, a smooth pebble, a velvety scarf. For each session, record the date, technique, location, and numerical intensity rating, along with a sentence or two about your accompanying emotional state.

At the end of each week, revisit both your journal and your body outline. Redraw the zones, adjusting color intensity or shape according to your newest findings. Perhaps the lower abdomen, once bathed in soft yellow, now deserves a richer orange hue after repeated reports of stronger sensations. Or maybe you discover an entirely new hotspot—behind the knees, on the upper arms— that was overlooked on your first tour. By iteratively refining the map in synchronization with your experiments, you transform it from a static snapshot into a responsive tool that reflects your evolving awareness.

It is crucial to approach this cycle with curiosity rather than judgment. Some sessions may feel uneventful; regions you expected to respond may lie dormant, while other areas surprise you with unexpected liveliness. That is precisely the point: the pleasure map is yours alone, unbound by norms or expectations. If an area persistently resists sensation, you might explore alternative prompts—changing the timing of your session, experimenting with different speeds of movement, or simply allowing more time for the nervous system to settle into a receptive mode. Conversely, if a particular technique yields consistently high ratings, you can earmark that region or method for deeper exploration in future cycles.

By the end of six weeks, you will have completed roughly half a dozen iterations of mapping, experimenting, and revising. The resulting blueprint will display a rich tapestry of zones and flows—some boldly highlighted, others softly shaded—together charting the unique geography of your pleasurable self. With this map in hand, you gain several practical advantages. First, you know where to direct your attention when you have limited time or energy—no more guessing at which regions might awaken your nervous system most gently or intensely. Second, you possess a clear record of what contexts and modalities tend to heighten your sensitivity, whether it is the warmth of morning light on the skin, the rhythmic pulse of breathwork, or the textured glide of a silk scarf. Finally, you cultivate a more nuanced relationship with your body's feedback loops, learning to trust the signals of tension and release, arousal and relaxation.

Beyond the six-week cycle, your pleasure map remains a living document. Life circumstances change: stress levels fluctuate, hormonal patterns shift, environmental stimuli vary with the seasons. Scheduling periodic reviews—perhaps quarterly or in alignment with your menstrual cycle—ensures that the map stays attuned to your present reality. Use each review as an opportunity to integrate new discoveries: perhaps partner experiences suggest fresh possibilities, or a new form of movement practice reveals hidden resonances. Over months and years, you will witness your pleasure map evolve into an intricate atlas of self-knowledge— one that not only supports more consistent satisfaction but also deepens your broader sense of embodiment and agency.

In sum, creating a personal pleasure map is less about crafting a perfect final artifact and more about engaging in a process of discovery. Structured journaling anchors your reflections in specific, recallable details. Visual mapping translates those details into a spatial language, revealing clusters of sensitivity and streams of energetic flow. Iterative refinement through focused experimentation turns insight into embodied skill, allowing you to navigate with precision through the landscape of your own pleasure. Equipped with these tools, you step into a more empowered relationship with your body—one that celebrates curiosity, honors individual variation, and recognizes pleasure as an integral dimension of holistic wellbeing. In the forthcoming sections, we will build upon this foundation to explore sensory layering, cultural scripts, and the psychological reframing needed to dissolve barriers to full, unabashed enjoyment.

2.2 Sensory Exploration Techniques

Exploring the senses offers a pathway into deeper awareness of the body's responses, helping to dismantle rote patterns of arousal and inviting fresh discovery. One accessible entry point is temperature variation. Imagine first trailing a length of cool silk across the skin of the forearm, noting the slight shiver it elicits as nerve endings awaken to the gentle chill. After this initial pass, warm a small glass bottle of oil between your palms until it feels comfortably tepid, then allow the oil to pool in your warm hand before pressing it onto the same patch of skin. The contrast between cool and warm—first the subtle nip of silk, then the enveloping embrace of oil—magnifies each sensation, pulling the nervous system's attention outward toward the borders of the body. As awareness heightens, the simplest shifts in temperature can feel enlivening rather than merely neutral. Over time, you may discover that alternating warm and cool touch in a steady rhythm produces a pleasurable crescendo, as though the skin itself were composing a melody of sensation.

Texture, too, holds transformative power. Feathers, with their gossamer softness, can trace barely perceptible currents of pleasure along the collarbone or the inner wrist, stirring dormant sensibilities in places rarely touched with such delicacy. A gentle brushing with a soft paintbrush across the lips or the back of the neck imparts a surprising intimacy, inviting the mind to focus wholly on the fleeting caress. Personal massage tools—whether a small handheld vibrator or a rolling massage ball—offer a different quality of feedback, blending steady pressure with rhythmic pulses. In experimenting with these implements, one might begin by simply holding each device against the skin without movement, noting its vibration frequency or the texture of its surface, then gradually increasing motion or pressure in accordance with the body's cues. By assigning a simple rating scale—perhaps mentally scoring each texture from one to ten based on ease of relaxation or intensity of sensation—you cultivate an empirical sense of what materials and modalities resonate most deeply with your unique somatic profile.

The richness of these explorations multiplies when senses are combined. In a session designed for multisensory layering, you might begin with a brief breathing exercise to center the mind, then select a signature scent—perhaps an essential oil of lavender for calm or a subtly sweet rosewater mist. As the aroma fills the room, you introduce a soundtrack: the gentle lap of ocean waves, the rustle of autumn leaves, or a piece of instrumental music that evokes expansiveness. With the olfactory and auditory environment established, you proceed to touch: first the cool silk, then the warmed oil, tracing paths that felt most potent during earlier experiments. As each layer overlaps, the brain's sensory centers engage in a richer dialogue, weaving together memory, emotion, and tactile awareness. This orchestration of scent, sound, and touch can amplify baseline sensitivity, making spatial gradients of temperature and texture feel more pronounced than when experienced in isolation. Over successive sessions, you learn not only which combinations evoke the most vivid responses, but also how to pace progression—beginning with subtler stimuli and advancing toward more pronounced contrasts as the nervous system grows accustomed to attentive exploration.

These sensory techniques do more than kindle momentary pleasure; they cultivate sustained interoceptive awareness. By repeatedly directing attention to subtle shifts in sensation, you strengthen the neural pathways that link external stimulus to internal experience. This process mirrors early developmental stages, when infants learn the world at the pace of touch, taste, sound, and smell. In adulthood, returning to that childlike curiosity—exploring textures and temperatures without expectation or goal—fosters a deeper connection to the body's aliveness. With practice, you begin to recognize cascading patterns: how a cool whisper of silk may lead to a sudden warmth around the spine, or how a particular vibration frequency encourages a release of tightness in the jaw. In this way, sensory exploration becomes both a method of discovery and a language of attunement, empowering you to communicate your needs more clearly to yourself and, if desired, to a partner.

2.3 Overcoming Cultural & Psychological Barriers

Even the most finely tuned sensory skills can be muted by invisible scripts that shape how we perceive our own bodies and desires. From early childhood, many of us absorb messages—through family attitudes, religious teachings, media portrayals, and peer commentary—that frame certain areas of touch as unseemly, certain expressions of pleasure as selfish or shameful. These internalized narratives, or "pleasure scripts," often operate below conscious awareness, pressing the brakes on exploration at the first hint of deviation from what feels "proper." Recognizing and dismantling these scripts is a vital step toward reclaiming agency over one's intimate life.

Identifying the contours of these scripts requires honest self-reflection. You may notice, upon closer examination, a twinge of discomfort when recalling a memory of playful tickling as a child, or an uneasy feeling when encountering media images that present sexuality as either exclusively youthful or grotesquely sensationalized. Perhaps family dynamics taught you that discussing bodily sensations was taboo, or religious doctrines instilled a belief that bodily pleasure is a distraction from spiritual pursuit. These messages imprint upon the neural circuits of the brain in the form of limiting beliefs: that your body is inherently flawed, that seeking pleasure equates to a lack of self-control, or that certain parts of your anatomy are off-limits to your own touch. By naming these scripts—writing sentences such as "I must be modest and not focus on my own pleasure" or "Expressing desire will make me selfish"—you bring implicit biases into the domain of explicit awareness, where they can be examined rather than allowed to govern unconsciously.

Once these limiting beliefs are surfaced, the work of cognitive restructuring can begin. Rather than attempting to shatter deep-seated convictions through sheer willpower, cognitive reframing invites gentle inquiry: What evidence supports this belief? What evidence contradicts it? If you held this belief twenty years from now, how might it look in hindsight? Through guided journaling exercises, you challenge automatic thoughts by reimagining them in more curious, compassionate language—transforming "I should feel ashamed when I touch myself" into "I am learning to honor my body's needs and signals." This process resembles the method used in cognitive behavioral therapy, where the interplay between thoughts, feelings, and behaviors is laid bare, allowing new, more supportive thought patterns to emerge. Over time, consistently practicing reframing nurtures a neuroplastic shift, weakening the old inhibitory circuits and strengthening pathways aligned with self-validation and exploration.

Complementing individual cognitive work, peer support and safe circles provide an invaluable container for normalization and growth. Participating in a group of trusted individuals—whether in a workshop setting led by a trained facilitator or an informal gathering of close friends—creates an environment where diverse experiences of pleasure can be shared without fear of judgment. Within these circles, each member has the opportunity to tell their story: recalling moments of awakening, confessing areas of lingering shame, asking questions that might feel too exposing in other contexts. The simple act of listening to another person's journey often stirs recognition of shared themes and validates one's own struggles or triumphs. Group practices may include guided sharing sessions, paired exercises such as mirror work with verbal affirmations, or co-created rituals around breath and movement. In witnessing others reclaim ownership of their bodies and desires, participants find permission to do the same for themselves.

Overcoming cultural and psychological barriers is neither a linear process nor a short-term project. You might find yourself revisiting certain scripts when life stress intensifies or new relational dynamics emerge. In those moments, the tools of naming limiting beliefs, reframing thoughts, and seeking communal support prove their lasting worth. As cognitive and social landscapes shift, you will notice that sensory exploration— once fraught with hesitation—flows more freely, unencumbered by shadowy doubts about legitimacy or worth. The body, which may once have felt foreign or overly regulated, becomes a trusted ally, guiding you toward experiences that reflect not inherited mandates, but your own authentic preferences. Ultimately, dismantling these barriers transforms pleasure from a seldom-visited curiosity into a natural continuum of wellbeing, integrated into the broader tapestry of life's richness.

Chapter 3: Communication, Consent & Negotiation

Research shows that couples who practice explicit consent models report 60% higher relationship satisfaction—an affirmation that clarity and mutual understanding do more than prevent boundary violations; they actively enhance intimacy, trust, and emotional safety. At its core, consent is not a one-time checkbox but an ongoing dialogue in which both partners continually express needs, desires, and limits. In this chapter, we explore the subtle choreography of giving and receiving consent, beginning with the dual channels of verbal agreement and non-verbal cues. By mastering the art of clear communication—through simple frameworks, attentive body-language decoding, and personalized signaling systems—you and your partner can navigate moments of closeness with confidence, respect, and genuine enthusiasm.

3.1 Verbal & Non-Verbal Consent Cues

Consent is most robust when it is explicit, enthusiastic, and ongoing. Yet many people struggle to articulate their comfort levels or to interpret a partner's signals without resorting to guesswork. The "Yes/No/Maybe" framework offers a user-friendly structure for turning desire discussions into straightforward conversations. At its simplest, a "yes" indicates clear enthusiasm, a "no" establishes a firm boundary, and a "maybe" invites further exploration or negotiation. Picture this exchange: one partner leans in and asks, "Would you like me to kiss you here?" A confident "yes" means proceed; a "no" means withdraw immediately; a "maybe" opens the door to clarification—"I'm not sure yet, could we start with gentler pressure?"

In practice, these verbal scripts can be woven seamlessly into intimate moments. Early on in a date, one might say, "I really enjoy holding your hand—does that feel comfortable?" eliciting a simple "yes" or "no," or perhaps a "I'd prefer if we keep our hands to ourselves for now." As attraction builds, the same framework applies to deeper forms of touch. A partner might pause and ask, "I'd like to explore more of your back with my fingertips—does that sound good?" If the response is "yes, please," momentum continues; if "no, thank you," attention shifts elsewhere; if "maybe later," the question transforms into a planning prompt: "When do you think you might feel ready?"

Crucially, the "maybe" category legitimizes ambivalence. Rather than evoking guilt or pressure, "maybe" signals a desire to learn more—either about what exactly is being offered or about one's own evolving comfort. It prevents consent from becoming binary and inflexible, allowing partners to chart a course toward mutual satisfaction while honoring each person's pace. Over time, using these simple verbal tools normalizes consent as a vital element of emotional attunement, rather than an awkward hurdle to overcome.

Yet words alone cannot carry the full weight of consent. Non-verbal communication often speaks more truthfully about our levels of comfort and engagement. Body language decoding begins with noticing the subtle physical shifts that accompany various emotional states. When someone feels safe and eager, their posture opens: shoulders relax, chest broadens, and the torso may lean forward. Eyes soften, pupils dilate, and breathing deepens. A partner who is genuinely interested may mirror your movements, nodding in rhythm with your words or gestures.

Conversely, hesitation often manifests as a slight recoil—a backward shift of the hips, a subtle lifting of the shoulders, or a momentary freeze in facial expression. The hands may tighten into gentle fists, or the legs may cross defensively under the table. Breathing may become shallow, and eye contact may flicker away. Recognizing these cues requires a foundation of presence: slowing down long enough to observe micro-movements and trusting your intuition if something feels off. If you notice a partner's chest rising and falling more quickly, or their gaze darting away, it can signal nervousness or uncertainty. Rather than assuming consent, you might pause and say, "I feel you're pulling back—would you like me to stop or check in?"

In addition to these spontaneous gestures, intentional non-verbal signals—safe words and bespoke systems—can further strengthen consent practices. A safe word is a pre-agreed term that, when spoken, immediately halts any activity. The ideal safe word is unlikely to arise in regular conversation—something like "pineapple" or "emerald." In moments of intensity, partners simply need to utter this word to draw an immediate, unquestioned boundary. Safe signals, meanwhile, can be silent gestures—pressing a single hand into the other's arm, tapping a thigh twice, or raising a palm. These non-verbal cues prove invaluable when speech fails—during moments of heavy breathing, overwhelming sensation, or if one partner's voice is soft or muffled.

Designing a personalized system of verbal and non-verbal signals begins with an open conversation outside of intimate contexts. Partners might sit together with tea or in a relaxed setting and outline which words or gestures feel most comfortable and memorable. They might practice role-playing scenarios: "What if I become too aroused to speak clearly—how would you prefer I signal a pause?" One partner could demonstrate exaggerating a hesitation gesture, and the other could respond with an example of pausing and checking in. Through these rehearsals, both people internalize the fluidity of consent, preparing for situations in which clear communication may otherwise be compromised.

An advanced application of this system is the integration of consent "checkpoints" throughout an experience. Instead of assuming passive continuation, partners agree to pause at set moments—after a certain number of kisses, or before moving from one type of touch to another—and to use the Yes/No/Maybe framework afresh. This ritualized approach ensures that consent remains an active dialogue, preventing situations where one partner "forgets" to ask or the other partner hesitates to speak up. It also models the idea that consent evolves with context: an enthusiastic "yes" to gentle stroking does not automatically extend to more intense forms of intimacy. By embedding checkpoints, partners reaffirm boundaries and desires continuously.

Throughout all of this, the tone of consent conversations matters as much as the words or signals themselves. When questions are asked with genuine curiosity and tenderness—rather than as perfunctory tasks—they invite honest responses. A soft voice, attentive eye contact, and an open posture convey respect and interest. Conversely, rushing through consent prompts or treating them as a mere formality can undermine trust. Partners should strive to create a container of emotional safety, where curiosity about each other's experiences is met with non-judgment and care.

It is also essential to recognize that consent is not only about preventing harm but about co-creating pleasure. Framing consent as a collaborative exploration—an opportunity to discover what feels good together—infuses it with positive energy. Phrases like "I want to know what brings you joy" or "Tell me how I can support your comfort" position consent as an affirmative force, rather than a defensive posture. When partners share enthusiasm for each other's responses, celebrating the vulnerability it takes to speak up, they build a climate where honest communication feels rewarding rather than risky.

Moreover, as relationships mature and circumstances shift— whether due to stress, illness, fatigue, or simply the ebb and flow of desire—consent practices must adapt. A "yes" given in one season of life may become a "maybe" or a "no" in another. Partners attuned to each other will notice these shifts and update their mutual agreements accordingly. Regular check-ins, perhaps at the end of a week or before an extended period apart, help ensure that consent practices remain aligned with each individual's current needs and boundaries.

In summary, mastering verbal and non-verbal consent cues transforms intimate encounters into acts of shared authorship. By employing the Yes/No/Maybe framework, partners gain a simple yet powerful script for expressing willingness and limits. By tuning into body language, they learn to see beneath the surface of words, catching hesitation or enthusiasm in the subtlest of gestures. And by designing safe words and signals, they safeguard communication even when speech falters. All of these elements coalesce into a living, responsive system that honors autonomy, fosters trust, and elevates pleasure through mutual respect. As you integrate these principles, consent ceases to be a barrier and instead becomes the very conduit through which deeper connection and authentic negotiation emerge. In the next section, we will build upon this foundation by exploring advanced communication models—tools for navigating more complex emotional terrain with empathy and clarity.

3.2 Advanced Communication Models

Beyond the foundational clarity of yes, no, and maybe, deeper emotional attunement often requires a more nuanced language—one that honors our inner needs without slipping into blame or defensiveness. Nonviolent Communication (NVC), developed by psychologist Marshall Rosenberg, offers a gentle yet powerful framework for this work. At its heart, NVC invites us first to observe concrete behaviors without judgment, then to name the feelings those behaviors evoke, to identify the underlying needs connected to those feelings, and finally to make a clear request. In intimate contexts, this four-step sequence transforms potentially fraught conversations into invitations for mutual understanding.

Imagine a scenario in which one partner feels overlooked when plans are made without their input. Rather than accusing—"You never ask me what I want; you're so selfish"—the NVC approach begins with a simple, objective observation: "Last week, when our weekend plans were finalized without checking in with me..." This moment of neutral description prevents defensive reactions by focusing on actions rather than character. The speaker then names their emotional response: "...I felt disappointed and a bit hurt..." By articulating feelings, the conversation shifts from attack-and-defend to an empathic exchange: "I felt disappointed and a bit hurt." Next comes the identification of needs: "...because I really value feeling seen and included when making decisions that affect both of us." In this way, the speaker connects their personal experience to a universal human need—inclusion and consideration—rather than making the partner responsible for their feelings. Finally, the request: "Would you be willing to discuss upcoming weekend plans with me before finalizing them?"

This sequence—observation, feeling, need, request—can be woven into moments of intimacy just as easily as into logistical conversations. Suppose one partner notices the other tense up whenever physical closeness shifts into more passionate touch. Rather than interpreting that tension as rejection or assuming blame, an NVC-informed approach might sound like this: "When you gently pull away after I kiss your neck (observation), I feel uncertain and a bit self-conscious (feeling), because I need to know that I'm attentive to your comfort levels (need). Would you be open to telling me what pace feels best for you right now?" This gentle inquiry both validates the partner's boundaries and creates space for honest feedback, strengthening trust rather than letting unspoken tension accumulate.

A related tool—often taught alongside NVC—is the simple "I feel... when you... because..." template. While it mirrors the NVC structure, its straightforward phrasing can feel more approachable in the heat of the moment. For instance: "I feel anxious when you look at your phone during our time together because I need to feel like I have your undivided attention." Or, in an affectionate context: "I feel cherished when you hold my hand on the walk home because it tells me you enjoy being close to me." By consistently using this template, couples replace vague complaints or passive-aggressive comments with precise emotional statements. The partner hearing these phrases is more likely to respond with empathy rather than defensiveness, because the focus remains on the speaker's internal experience rather than faulting the other person.

While it can feel awkward at first to voice these structured statements, practicing them in writing can build confidence and fluency. Journal-based role-play offers a safe rehearsal space. Begin by selecting a challenging conversation you anticipate— for example, a need for more frequent check-ins or a wish to experiment with new forms of closeness. In your journal, write a script in which you play both roles, alternating between "Speaker" and "Listener." As the Speaker, draft your observation, feeling, need, and request, then switch hats and craft the Listener's empathic response: perhaps a validating acknowledgment and an offer to discuss solutions. After drafting, reflect on any words or tones that feel awkward or overly formal, and revise until the language sounds natural and caring.

Next, imagine the real-life context: Where will you have this talk? Sitting in the living room at a calm moment, over tea before bedtime, or on a leisurely Sunday morning? Visualizing the scene helps integrate the language into your bodily sense of safety, so that when the moment arrives, you are less likely to freeze or revert to old patterns. Some people also find it helpful to read their scripted lines aloud into a voice memo, then listen back to gauge the emotional tone. Through these journal-based rehearsals, you cultivate a kind of muscle memory for compassionate communication. By the time you bring the conversation into the living room, both your mind and body carry a sense of readiness.

Importantly, advanced communication models like NVC are not rigid formulas but living guidelines. In real-time, you may not recall the four words "observation, feeling, need, request," yet the practiced rhythm of noticing, naming, and inviting helps conversations stay anchored in empathy. Over weeks and months, as you and your partner integrate these tools, you will likely notice fewer misunderstandings, more ease in discussing sensitive topics, and an emerging culture of curiosity—where both people feel heard, valued, and motivated to seek win-win solutions.

3.3 Digital Tools & Tracking Boundaries

In our digitally connected age, communication and consent need not be confined to face-to-face moments alone. A growing ecosystem of apps and devices can support shared understanding of desires, boundaries, and emotional needs—provided they are used thoughtfully, transparently, and with respect for privacy.

One popular category of applications centers on shared desire calendars and boundary logs. These tools allow partners to schedule time for intimacy in advance—whether that means setting aside a weekday evening for a date night or noting a weekend morning for shared quiet time. Beyond simple calendar functions, many apps offer customizable tags or color codes to indicate preferred types of connection—for instance, "cuddle," "conversation," or "sensual massage." Users can also log boundaries: marking days when they feel low energy and might need space, or indicating specific topics or actions they wish to postpone. Having these preferences recorded in a shared digital space ensures that each partner's needs are visible without assumptions.

When choosing such an app, privacy considerations are paramount. Ideally, the tool should offer end-to-end encryption so that only you and your partner can read entries. Local data storage—keeping logs on your own device rather than in a central server—further minimizes risk. Look for options to password-protect the app or to hide it behind a discreet icon, respecting the fact that personal notes about intimacy may feel sensitive. Customization features—such as adding your own mood tags or boundary descriptors—allow the app to grow with your relationship, rather than forcing you into predefined categories.

For those who wish to incorporate physiological feedback into their understanding of readiness and boundaries, wearable technology offers new possibilities. Smart rings, fitness trackers, and smartwatches can continuously monitor metrics such as heart rate, heart rate variability (HRV), skin temperature, and even sleep patterns. By sharing selected data streams—always by mutual consent—partners can gain insights into each other's stress levels and physiological arousal. For example, a partner might notice elevated heart rate and shallow breathing during a busy workday, signaling a need for calm rather than intimacy. Conversely, a pattern of rising HRV in the evening could indicate a window of lower stress and greater receptivity.

Yet with this power comes responsibility. Any bio-data sharing agreement must begin with a clear conversation about which metrics will be shared, how often, and through what channels. Partners should establish protocols for interpreting the data— avoiding assumptions that a high heart rate automatically means sexual arousal or that a low skin temperature signals disinterest. Both parties must retain the right to pause or revoke data sharing at any time. Ethical use of wearable feedback hinges on ongoing dialogue: checking in about how the data feels to both people, and ensuring it enhances understanding rather than eroding trust or fostering surveillance.

Finally, digital tools can also help automate reminders and check-ins to reassess consent over time. Instead of relying on memory or letting discussions slide when life gets hectic, partners can schedule recurring prompts—weekly, biweekly, or monthly— asking questions like "How have you felt about our recent intimacy?" or "Is there anything you'd like to try or discuss this month?" These automated touchpoints, delivered by text message or app notification, reduce the burden of initiating delicate topics. They turn boundary discussions into routine practice rather than crisis interventions. To prevent these reminders from becoming burdensome, it's wise to allow for easy rescheduling, silencing, or deferral—acknowledging that emotional bandwidth fluctuates.

When combined, shared calendars, wearable feedback, and automated reminders form a digital scaffold that supports ongoing consent and connection. But technology should never replace empathetic, in-person conversations; rather, it should augment them. After a period of digital data collection—perhaps two months of calendar logs, mood tags, and HRV readings—set aside time to sit together, review the patterns, and discuss any surprises. Translate numbers and tags into lived experience: What did it feel like when intimacy was scheduled versus spontaneous? How did your moods align or diverge? What unspoken needs surfaced through the data? In this way, digital tools become a bridge between quantitative insights and qualitative dialogues, reinforcing the trust that lays the groundwork for enduring intimacy.

By thoughtfully integrating advanced communication models, personalized consent rituals, and supportive digital systems, couples can create a rich ecosystem of clarity and care. Each element—from the precise language of NVC to the discreet logs in a shared app—strengthens the scaffolding of mutual respect. Over time, these practices foster an environment in which desires, boundaries, and emotional currents flow freely between partners, cultivating healthier, more satisfying connections.

Chapter 4: Emotional Intimacy & Attachment Styles

Securely attached women report twice the sexual satisfaction compared to those with anxious or avoidant attachments—a striking testament to the power of emotional safety in the bedroom and beyond. Understanding how attachment patterns shape our capacity for closeness is not an abstract psychological exercise but a practical step toward deeper intimacy, greater confidence, and an enriched love life. In this section, we guide you through three essential phases: discovering your own attachment style through reliable self-assessment quizzes; tracing its roots back to early family dynamics and the stories you learned about love; and crafting a personalized action plan to cultivate secure attachment behaviors that nourish both your relationships and your sexual wellbeing.

4.1 Identifying Your Attachment Patterns

To begin, imagine attachment styles not as rigid categories but as fluid tendencies—habits of relating that develop from infancy and continue to influence how you seek comfort, express desire, and respond to closeness. The four primary attachment frameworks—secure, anxious, avoidant, and disorganized—offer a map for recognizing patterns that may otherwise feel confusing or shame-laden. Secure attachment is marked by comfort with both independence and intimacy; anxious attachment often shows up as worry about abandonment; avoidant attachment manifests as discomfort with closeness or a habit of emotional withdrawal; and disorganized attachment can appear as a perplexing mix of anxiety and avoidance, sometimes triggered by trauma.

Reliable self-assessment quizzes serve as a convenient first step in clarifying where you fall on this spectrum. Conducted in a quiet moment, these quizzes usually consist of statements such as "I find it easy to trust my partner" or "I often worry that I am not lovable." Rather than taking any single question as definitive, the quizzes aggregate responses across multiple dimensions—your comfort with intimacy, your anxiety about rejection, and your reliance on self-sufficiency. Online tools created by attachment researchers or reputable relationship coaches can guide you, but you may also craft your own assessment by listing twenty to thirty reflective statements and rating how much each resonates on a scale from "strongly disagree" to "strongly agree." To interpret your results, look for clusters: if most of your high scores indicate tension around closeness and fear of abandonment, you may lean toward an anxious style; if high marks align with reluctance to depend on others, you may lean toward avoidance. A balance of positive affirmations around trust, flexibility, and comfort with intimacy suggests secure attachment, whereas inconsistent or extreme responses across categories may point to a disorganized pattern.

However, quizzes alone cannot tell the full story. The numerical snapshot they provide gains depth when you reflect on concrete relational experiences. Think back to a time when you felt emotionally overwhelmed—perhaps you became angry or anxious when a partner did not return your calls, or withdrew entirely when conflict arose. Write about the sensations in your body, the inner dialogue that unfolded, and the actions you took. Did you send repeated messages pleading for reassurance? Did you freeze and refuse to engage further? Juxtapose these accounts with memories of feeling safe and supported—moments when honest conversations flowed easily, when you could express desire without fear of judgment. These written reflections complement your quiz results and begin to illuminate the patterns that recur across different relationships and life stages.

To understand how these styles originate, we turn our gaze to the root causes embedded in early family dynamics. Attachment patterns are shaped during infancy and childhood, as primary caregivers respond—or fail to respond—to a child's emotional and physical needs. When a caregiver consistently meets a baby's hunger cues, soothes distress, and provides predictable comfort, the child learns that the world is a safe place and that it is permissible to depend on others. This foundation fosters secure attachment, visible in adulthood as an ability to communicate needs, to regulate emotions, and to trust a partner's intentions.

In contrast, anxious attachment often takes root when caregiving is inconsistent—sometimes warm and attentive, sometimes distant or preoccupied. A child learns that love is unpredictable, and so grows up perpetually vigilant: watching for signs of rejection, seeking frequent reassurance, and fearing abandonment. As an adult, this translates into heightened sensitivity to perceived slights, a tendency to seek overreassurance, and an emotional roller coaster driven by fear more than desire.

Avoidant attachment, on the other hand, often emerges when caregivers regularly rebuff the child's bids for comfort—dismissing tears, encouraging early self-soothing, or emphasizing independence above emotional expression. The child learns that needs are best buried rather than voiced. In adult relationships, this can show up as a reluctance to share feelings, a preference for emotional distance, and even a judgment that intimacy itself is a form of weakness.

A disorganized attachment style develops in the context of frightening or traumatic caregiving—when the person charged with protection also becomes a source of threat or confusion. This can occur in homes marked by abuse, neglect, or severe parental dysregulation. The child's survival strategy becomes a chaotic mix of approach and avoidance, never fully trusting or fully rejecting the caregiver. In adult intimacy, this disorganized pattern may manifest as unpredictable swings between clinging and pushing away, a profound inner conflict that can leave both partners bewildered.

To trace your own roots, revisit key memories from your childhood with journal prompts designed for depth rather than breadth. Describe your earliest recollection of feeling upset and how comfort arrived or failed to arrive. Note how affection was shown in your family—through words, hugs, or the absence of physical touch. Reflect on mealtime dynamics, bedtime routines, and the emotional availability of caregivers: was there space for tears and questions, or did you learn to stifle both? Although memories can be selective, patterns often emerge across different episodes, painting a coherent picture of the relational climate in which your attachment style first took shape.

Once you have mapped your style and surveyed its origins, the final step in this section is to develop a personalized action plan for moving toward secure attachment behaviors. Secure attachment does not require perfection; rather, it involves learning to balance autonomy with closeness, to communicate needs clearly, and to tolerate uncertainty without panic. For someone with an anxious tendency, the plan might include practices that build internal steadiness: daily journaling exercises that cultivate self-compassion, mindfulness meditations that anchor attention in the present rather than fixating on imagined rejection, and regular check-ins with a trusted friend or therapist to process fears before they escalate.

If avoidance is your default, you might begin by deliberately practicing small acts of vulnerability—sending a message that expresses a mild preference, such as "I'd love to hear your thoughts about our plan for this weekend," and observing the outcome. Over time, these micro-disclosures—sharing a fleeting irritation or a moment of loneliness—loosely approximate the experience of emotional risk, gradually desensitizing the aversion to intimacy. You might also schedule weekly "connection appointments" during which you commit to sharing an honest feeling or asking for what you need, whether or not the mood feels perfect.

For those who recognize a disorganized pattern, an effective action plan often entails a combination of the techniques above, supplemented by trauma-informed support. Somatic therapies—such as gentle breathwork, body-oriented counseling, or sensorimotor psychotherapy—can help regulate the nervous system's inconsistent responses to closeness. Partnered exercises in attunement, where you practice tracking each other's emotional states in a safe, structured dialogue, can provide corrective relational experiences that rewire the disorganized pattern toward coherence.

Regardless of where you begin, three core principles should guide your action plan. First, cultivate awareness without judgment. Observe your instinctive reactions in moments of intimacy—as you would watch weather patterns—without labeling yourself good or bad. Second, advance in small, manageable steps. Radical change rarely happens overnight; instead, focus on incremental shifts, like pausing before responding when you feel anxious or intentionally leaning in when you feel the urge to pull away. Third, seek supportive relationships. Whether through therapy, friendship, or peer groups, having a trusted container in which to practice new behaviors accelerates the journey toward secure attachment.

In implementing these strategies, track your progress as you did with your initial quizzes. Revisit your self-assessment tool after six weeks, noting any shifts in your scores toward security.

Journal about landmark moments—times when you expressed a need and had it met, or when you tolerated uncertainty without spiraling into anxiety. Celebrate these successes as evidence that new neural pathways are forming; secure attachment is not an innate gift but a skill that can be cultivated, practiced, and mastered.

By identifying your attachment patterns, understanding their origins, and engaging in targeted exercises, you lay the groundwork for a relational transformation. No matter where you begin—anxiety, avoidance, or the disarray of mixed signals—moving toward secure attachment unlocks a reservoir of trust, closeness, and emotional freedom. These qualities are the bedrock of satisfying sexual experiences and the glue that binds loving partnerships. As you continue through this handbook, carry forward the insights of this section: that your attachment story, while powerful, is not fixed. With intention, compassion, and practice, you can rewrite old scripts and build the secure foundation upon which lasting intimacy thrives.

4.2 Rituals for Deep Vulnerability

True emotional intimacy thrives in the fertile ground of vulnerability, where partners meet not only in shared joy but also in mutual surrender to uncertainty. Rituals designed to cultivate and honor that vulnerability provide a structured path toward deeper connection, reminding each person that exposure of the heart is met with care rather than judgment. One powerful exercise begins with mirror gazing: partners sit facing each other, at a distance that allows eye contact without tension, and simply hold each other's gaze for several minutes. At first, the act may feel awkward, even exposing, as familiar defenses arise—the urge to break eye contact, to look away at a distraction. Yet as the silence stretches, the subtle nuances of the other's expression become luminous: a softened brow, the gentle rise and fall of breath, the light that flickers in their pupils at the moment of recognition. This shared stillness cultivates an implicit message: here we are, fully seen, without need for words or performance.

Building on the stillness of mirror gazing, synchronized breathing leads partners into a form of physiological attunement. After concluding the silent gaze, they turn slightly toward one another, each placing a hand over their own heart. Together, they begin to inhale deeply through the nose for a count of four, hold briefly, and exhale slowly through the mouth for a count of six. As their breath cycles align, the quality of the shared space shifts: heart rates settle into parallel rhythms, and the vagus nerve—pulling double duty as the body's "social engagement" highway—becomes more active. In this state of co-regulation, anxiety loosens its grip and the nervous system opens to the possibility of tenderness. Partners may choose to maintain eye contact through the breathing exercise, or to close their eyes, allowing the sense of presence to be felt inwardly. Either way, the mutual stillness reinforces the unspoken promise: I am here with you, safe and steady.

Empathic listening rounds out these shared vulnerability practices by offering a sacred container for each person's inner world. In empathic listening, one partner speaks for a set span of time—perhaps three to five minutes—sharing a current fear, a longing, or a fragment of vulnerability without fear of interruption. The listening partner's role is not to judge, to problem-solve, or to correct; rather, it is to reflect back what was heard, checking for accuracy and emotional resonance: "It sounds like you're feeling uncertain about our plans next week, and that makes you anxious because you need reassurance." This reflective approach acknowledges the speaker's experience as valid and real, weaving it into the relational fabric rather than brushing it aside. After the listener's reflection, the speaker may clarify or deepen the expression, and then roles reverse. Through this ritual, each person practices both courageous disclosure and gentle, compassionate reception. Over time, the pattern of empathic exchange deepens trust, showing that even the most tender admissions can land softly in the other's heart.

Beyond these formal exercises, gratitude and acknowledgment ceremonies create moments of shared celebration around the ongoing bravery of vulnerability. At a chosen cadence—weekly, biweekly, or monthly—partners come together in a dedicated space, perhaps lit by a single candle or infused with a favorite essential oil. Each takes a turn expressing gratitude for a specific act of courage the other displayed since the last ceremony: "I want to thank you for sharing your fear about your upcoming presentation; it helped me understand how to support you." The listener responds by acknowledging the impact of that courage: "Hearing your admission made me feel closer to you, and I appreciate your trust." These rituals need not be elaborate. A simple token—a small stone, a flower petal, or a written note—can serve as a physical reminder of the ceremony's intention, carried in a pocket or placed on the bedside table. The repeated rhythm of honoring vulnerability trains both partners' attention toward the strengths inherent in openness, rather than focusing solely on resolutions or achievements.

To weave vulnerability into daily life, micro-rituals offer bite-sized practices that sustain attunement even during busy weeks. One such ritual is the "rose, bud, thorn" check-in: each partner shares three brief reflections at a chosen moment—perhaps over morning coffee or during an evening walk. First, the "rose": a moment of joy or connection experienced that day. Second, the "bud": an emerging possibility or intention, such as a new idea for spending time together or a personal goal each is nurturing. Third, the "thorn": a difficulty or concern—a fleeting anxiety, a misunderstanding, or a physical ache in need of attention. By limiting each share to a few sentences, the ritual remains manageable, yet it fosters regular exchange of both positive and challenging experiences. Partners learn to listen without rushing to fix or minimize—the thorn is simply acknowledged, not immediately solved—reinforcing the lesson that vulnerability can coexist with everyday life, not only in grand moments of crisis or confession.

Over weeks and months, these rituals—mirror gazing, synchronized breathing, empathic listening, gratitude ceremonies, and rose/bud/thorn check-ins—form a constellation of practices that illuminate the terrain of vulnerability. They remind partners that exposing one's inner world is an act of intimacy rather than weakness, and that receiving another's truth with warmth rather than fear fosters deeper connection. As vulnerability becomes a shared practice, the scaffolding of trust grows sturdier, providing a secure foundation for the richer layers of emotional and sexual intimacy yet to come.

4.3 Healing Past Relationship Trauma

While vulnerability rituals build safety in the present, many women carry echoes of past wounds—moments when intimacy felt dangerous rather than nurturing. Healing these relational traumas is essential for reclaiming bodily autonomy and restoring the capacity to experience pleasure and closeness without fear. Somatic experiencing, a body-centered therapeutic method developed by Dr. Peter Levine, offers a step-by-step protocol for renegotiating bodily boundaries in the aftermath of sexual trauma. The process begins with titration—approaching traumatic sensations in minuscule, tolerable increments rather than attempting to confront the full intensity all at once. A facilitator might guide you to recall a distressing memory just enough to notice a mild physical sensation—perhaps a tightening in the chest or a flicker of heat. Rather than diving into the full emotional torrent, you pause and direct attention to a resource that feels safe—a warm blanket, a favorite song, or the sturdy presence of the therapist's hand on your arm. Through this pendulation—moving between the edges of discomfort and the refuge of safety—the nervous system learns that it can revisit difficult material without being overwhelmed.

As the process advances, the length of time spent near the traumatic edge gradually increases, and the supportive resources become internalized rather than external. You may practice co-regulating with a trusted partner or therapist at home, using shared breathing exercises to anchor the system once the memory arises. Over sessions, the body begins to renegotiate its physical boundaries: areas that once tensed reflexively—such as the pelvic region—learn to soften under voluntary control. By the end of the somatic experiencing sequence, many women report a newfound sense of ownership over their bodily responses—a confidence that the body will not be hijacked by past trauma but can instead be guided by present choice.

Eye Movement Desensitization and Reprocessing (EMDR) provides another powerful avenue for processing intimacy-related trauma. In EMDR, bilateral stimulation—through guided eye movements, tactile taps, or audio tones—accompanies focused work on distressing images or beliefs. Adapted for issues of sexual trust and desire, EMDR sessions might target core negative cognitions such as "I am not safe in my body" or "I am unworthy of pleasure." The therapist guides the client to hold these beliefs lightly in mind while tracking the bilateral stimulus, fostering rapid reprocessing that reduces the emotional charge of the memory. Following installation phases, patients often notice a shift in their bodily reactions: the sense of claustrophobia or dissociation that once accompanied intimacy weakens, making room for curiosity and willingness to experiment with closeness again.

Deciding between peer support groups and individual therapy—or choosing to combine both—depends on personal comfort, resources, and the nature of one's trauma. Peer support groups offer validation through shared narratives: hearing others articulate similar struggles can dissolve the isolation that often accompanies sexual trauma. Within a well-facilitated group, members take turns sharing and actively listening, providing mutual empathy and practical suggestions. The communal environment fosters solidarity and can spark inspiration for new coping strategies. However, group settings also carry risks: hearing others' detailed trauma stories may trigger secondary distress, and confidentiality concerns may surface if the group lacks strong agreements.

Individual therapy, in contrast, provides a private container tailored exclusively to your history and needs. A skilled clinician can pace interventions precisely, adjust modalities on the fly, and maintain strict confidentiality. The one-on-one relationship itself can become reparative—offering a corrective experience in which your boundaries are honored and your body's responses are treated with gentle curiosity. The drawback may be cost, limited availability, or the time required to build a therapeutic alliance.

Many women find that integrating both approaches yields the richest results. They attend a weekly support group for ongoing camaraderie and share generalized concerns, while simultaneously working in individual therapy on deeper, more personal material requiring professional discretion. Over months of combined engagement, skills learned in group—such as empathic listening—translate into richer therapeutic dialogues, while breakthroughs in individual sessions enhance the sense of safety and trust within the peer community.

Regardless of the path chosen, commitment to healing past relationship trauma is a profound act of self-respect. As body memories uncoil and cognitive reframing takes hold, you reclaim the autonomy to define your own boundaries, desires, and expressions of intimacy. The rituals of vulnerability discussed earlier become not only practices for the present moment but celebrations of the freedom won through courageous inner work. In this way, healing and vulnerability intertwine—each fueling the other in an upward spiral of trust, connection, and authentic expression.

Chapter 5: Body Positivity & Self-Image

5.1 Media Literacy & Deconstructing Beauty Myths

When the majority of women—an estimated eighty percent—report that dissatisfaction with their bodies undermines their confidence in intimate contexts, it becomes clear that our collective image of beauty exerts a profound influence on personal wellbeing. Yet beneath the glossy surfaces of magazines and the curated feeds of social media lies a world of digital manipulation, selective framing, and relentless algorithmic signals. To reclaim a sense of embodied self-love, it is essential first to develop media literacy: an ability to see through the artifice of "perfect" images and to understand how those images shape our own inner narratives. This journey begins with hands-on exploration of photo editing techniques, continues with a purposeful detox from comparison-driven platforms, and culminates in the curation of a feed that reflects the genuine diversity of human bodies and experiences.

Consider, for instance, the familiar sight of a fashion magazine spread: the model's waist seems impossibly narrow, the skin flawless, the lighting impeccable. What the eye perceives as natural beauty is often the result of layered interventions. In a workshop setting—whether in a community center, a classroom, or via a guided online tutorial—participants can learn to replicate these interventions on their own photographs. Opening an image in a common editing program, one first encounters the "liquify" tool, which subtly shifts contours: a ribcage drawn in, a torso elongated, hips smoothed into an hourglass shape. Highlighting and shadow adjustment tools paint on artificial depth, reinforcing the illusion of sculpted musculature or bone structure. Saturation sliders intensify skin tones, while blemishes are erased with a simple brushstroke. As participants apply these changes in real time, they witness how minor alterations—a fraction of a millimeter of warp here, a half-stop of brightness there—can transform an ordinary snapshot into an "ideal" portrait. This hands-on exercise demystifies the process and exposes the dissonance between reality and its representations. When we see how easily pixels can be molded to fit a narrow standard, we begin to question why we ever held ourselves to an unattainable blueprint.

Armed with this critical insight, the next step is to examine our daily media consumption habits. Many women find that even with a healthy skepticism about magazines, the steady stream of filtered selfies, influencer content, and targeted advertisements on social platforms continues to undermine self-image. A structured social media detox—a fourteen-day protocol—offers a reset, creating a window of freedom from relentless comparison. Day one might involve a complete unfollowing of accounts that consistently trigger negative self-judgment: influencers who represent a singular aesthetic or celebrities whose perfectly staged lives feel remote. Essential to the process is replacing these voids with neutral or positive accounts: perhaps a local gardening cooperative, a scientific news outlet, or the archive of a world-music radio station. Rather than leaving the space empty, one fills the feed with content that neither celebrates nor criticizes appearance, allowing the mind to shift its focus toward diverse interests. Over the course of the two weeks, participants gradually reintroduce only those accounts that contribute to learning, laughter, or a genuine sense of connection. By the end of the detox, the feed no longer feels like a hall of mirrors reflecting impossible ideals, but a tapestry of voices offering knowledge, inspiration, and authentic humanity.

Simultaneously, the detox process serves as a practice in mindfulness. Rather than succumbing to the habitual scroll, individuals are encouraged to pause and notice bodily sensations at moments of potential comparison: a tightening in the chest upon seeing a model's toned abs, a sinking in the gut at an influencer's flawless complexion. Recording these somatic reactions in a brief daily journal entry reinforces awareness of the emotional impact of curated images. Over time, the knots of comparison that once went unnoticed become clear signals to redirect attention toward more nourishing activities—reading a favorite book, taking a brisk walk, or calling a trusted friend.

With heightened discernment and a cleansed social feed, one can embark on the final phase of media literacy: curating a personalized stream of diverse, body-affirming role models. This involves an active search for creators and communities that celebrate the full spectrum of human form—women of different ages, ethnicities, abilities, and body types sharing unfiltered glimpses into their lives. A useful strategy is to seek out hashtags and online collectives dedicated to body positivity, intuitive movement, and authentic self-expression. When encountering a new account, one evaluates its content through the lens of impact: does it feel inviting and inclusive, offering stories of resilience, creativity, or joy? Or does it adhere to a narrow aesthetic that, while perhaps inspiring on one level, risks perpetuating old hierarchies of beauty? By gradually constructing a feed that features dancers with varied body types, writers exploring the intersection of culture and self-care, and photographers highlighting unretouched images, women can replace the linear narrative of "better, thinner, younger" with a kaleidoscope of expressions that validate their own unique worth.

As this curated environment takes shape, it becomes not only a source of visual pleasure but also a springboard for new learning. A dancer's slow-motion video can encourage viewers to appreciate the power of muscle engagement rather than its size.

A poet's reflection on aging may offer solace and wisdom, reminding readers that every line on the face carries a story of laughter or tears. A crafts collective's spotlight on people with disabilities underscores that beauty and capability coexist in manifold ways. Over time, these voices become internalized companions, guiding the mind away from automatic critiques and toward an expansive view of possible selves.

Critically, media literacy is not a one-and-done achievement but an ongoing practice. Just as the pernicious effects of edited images reassert themselves if one remains passive, so too must the commitment to seek and uplift positive representations be renewed periodically. Quarterly reviews of one's social feed, a return to photo-editing workshops, or the sharing of favorite body-affirming accounts with friends can reinforce the habits of discernment. In group settings, collective media-deconstruction sessions—where friends dissect a magazine spread or compare notes on digital detox experiences—nurture a culture of mutual support, multiplying the benefits beyond the individual.

Through this layered approach—understanding the mechanics of photo editing, detoxing from harmful digital influences, and curating a celebratory feed—women can dismantle the internalized myths of beauty that once dictated their self-perception. In doing so, they create fertile ground for "embodied self-love," a practice that sees the body not as a site of constant critique but as a wise, feeling instrument worthy of respect and care. Freed from the unrealistic standards of retouched images, each woman can begin to chart her own course toward confidence, presence, and authentic expression, laying the groundwork for the chapters that follow on movement, pleasure, and holistic wellbeing.

5.2 Embodied Self-Acceptance Practices

Learning to inhabit one's own body with kindness and curiosity often begins with the simple yet profound act of mirror work. This practice involves standing before a full-length mirror—ideally in a quiet, private space—and speaking aloud affirmations that gently challenge ingrained self-criticism. On the first day, you might begin with short, three-minute sessions focused simply on eye contact: looking into your own reflection and naming a single neutral observation, such as the color of your eyes or the shape of your collarbone. As the days progress, you gradually lengthen the duration and introduce affirmations that resonate with your personal journey: "I am learning to appreciate every curve that tells the story of my life," or "My body is a vessel of strength and compassion." The key is progression rather than perfection. By week two, sessions expand to ten minutes, allowing you to move from neutral observations into gentle praise for specific features that you may once have disparaged—a softly rounded belly that nourishes you, legs that carry you forward each day, hands that hold warmth for others. Each affirmation, spoken with deliberate intention, begins to rewire neural pathways of self-talk. Over time, mirror work shifts from a moment of anxiety to an act of self-honoring, rewiring the soundtrack in your mind from critique to compassion.

Yet mirror work is only one facet of embodied acceptance. Dance improvisation offers a dynamic avenue for celebrating the body in motion. Unlike choreographed routines, improvisational dance prizes spontaneity and playfulness. To get started, choose a piece of music that elicits joy—perhaps a rhythmic drumbeat or a soulful melody. Allow your eyes to close for a moment, sensing the music's pulse within your chest, and then open them and invite your body to respond. You might notice that your shoulders sway in time, that your hips tilt gently, or that your arms stretch toward the ceiling as if greeting the sky. Rather than judging each movement as "good" or "bad," simply honor its emergence. Guided prompts can enrich this process: imagine tracing the outline of a flower petal with your fingertips, or picture roots extending from your feet into the floor as you sway. These visualizations encourage you to explore different planes of movement, finding delight in the body's fluid capacities. As you move, pay attention to sensations—perhaps warmth pooling in the chest or a pleasurable tremor in the thighs. By the end of each session, take a moment to rest, placing a hand over your heart and acknowledging the vitality that arises when you dance without agenda. Repeated practice dissolves shame around movement and reveals the body as a source of joyful expression rather than performance.

Art therapy techniques provide another fertile ground for transforming body image narratives. Working with clay, for instance, invites tactile engagement that can bypass the often-critical internal voice. Begin by molding a simple form—perhaps a sphere or a cylinder—allowing the clay's cool resistance to remind you of your own physical presence. As you press and squeeze, notice any judgments that surface: "This clay feels too sticky," or "I cannot make it smooth enough." Acknowledge these thoughts, then shift attention to texture and shape, observing how the clay yields to intent. Gradually introduce more figurative work: sculpt a torso, paying attention to how your hands perceive curves and angles. Resist the urge to smooth away every imperfection; instead, let each indentation and ridge stand as a testament to authenticity. After a sculpting session, journal about what emerged—did the shoulders feel tense as you molded, or did the clay's pliability mirror your own flexibility?

If painting is more inviting, set up a simple art station with watercolors or acrylics. Select a warm, supportive palette—perhaps soft pinks, earth tones, and gentle blues—and let your brush move freely across the paper. You might begin with broad strokes that mimic the arch of a back or the curve of a hip, then layer in details that feel resonant: droplets of color that shimmer like light on skin or sweeping lines that trace out an arm in flight. Throughout the process, pay attention to the internal dialogue that arises. When the critic's voice whispers that your brushwork is "messy," pause and redirect your hand with curiosity: Why did it choose that shape? What story might it tell? By externalizing body image through art, you create a safe distance from internal judgments. The painting or sculpture becomes a mirror of your perceptions, allowing you to step back, reflect, and then re-engage with gentler self-observation.

Over weeks and months, these embodied self-acceptance practices weave together into a tapestry of profound transformation. Mirror work retrains the mind's voice; dance improvisation reawakens the body's intrinsic joy; art therapy externalizes and reframes long-held beliefs. As the practitioner moves through these modalities, a new relationship with the body emerges—one grounded not in aspiration toward external ideals but in celebration of personal experience, sensation, and creative expression. This reclaimed foundation of self-acceptance sets the stage for the next exploration, where fashion, movement, and self-expression merge to deepen confidence and presence in daily life.

5.3 Fashion, Movement & Erotic Self-Expression

Fashion can be a powerful ally in cultivating confidence and self-love. Clothing choices that once felt driven by trends or expectations can be reshaped into an intimate conversation between fabric, form, and personal narrative. Start by curating an "intimate wardrobe" that honors how you wish to feel—whether that is enveloped in softness, empowered by structure, or enlivened by vibrant color. Slip your hand over different fabrics and note how each sensation resonates against the skin. Perhaps a silk camisole evokes a sense of fluid elegance, its coolness following the line of the collarbone; or a high-waisted cotton skirt offers a gentle hug around the waist, affirming the body's curves with supportive embrace. By selecting garments that feel harmonious with your body's rhythms, you create a daily costume that reinforces self-acceptance rather than masking perceived flaws.

The process of wardrobe curation also involves experimenting with cuts and silhouettes that defy previous assumptions about what "flatters" your shape. Try a bias-cut dress that drapes diagonally across the torso, or a tailored blazer with pronounced shoulders that shift focus toward strength in posture. Notice how different pieces encourage you to move: a swing skirt may invite a playful twirl, while a pair of fitted trousers might prompt you to walk with deliberate stride. In each case, the mirror confirms not just how you appear but how you inhabit the clothes—an essential feedback loop that informs future selections. Over time, your wardrobe becomes an extension of your inner landscape, each outfit a reflection of your present mood and desired expression.

Movement practices such as slow-flow dance or introductory burlesque basics offer another dimension of self-expression. Slow-flow dance, inspired by yoga and contemporary dance, emphasizes the continuous transition from one shape to another. In a typical session, you move through a series of postures—arching, folding, spiraling—synchronized with breath. The dance unfolds not as a rigid sequence, but as a personalized exploration: you pause in a high lunge to feel the lengthening of the hip flexors, then let your torso spiral into a standing twist, letting arms float behind you as though painting arcs in the air. This unhurried pace allows full attention to the sensations in muscles, joints, and connective tissues, fostering a sense of embodiment that transcends aesthetics. The practice itself becomes an affirmation of the body's capacity to transform, flow, and adapt.

For those drawn to the theatrical flair of burlesque, basic techniques can be adapted to everyday self-expression. You might stand before a mirror and experiment with the arch of the back, placing one hand on the hip and the other tracing a sinuous line from the shoulder to the waist. A soft reframing of the movement—calling it "artistic expression" rather than "seduction"—helps maintain the practice within a self-affirming context. Incorporating a scarf or a feather boa adds a tactile dimension: the light brush of the feathers retraces the curves you have learned to celebrate in earlier mirror work sessions. Through these choreographed shapes, you train your body to command attention—to stand with presence and poise—whether or not you are performing for an audience. Even in solitary practice, the burlesque-inspired movements embed a newfound appreciation for the body's capacity to provoke emotion and convey confidence.

Accessorizing provides a final layer of empowerment, a way to punctuate your chosen aesthetic with meaningful details. Jewelry—whether a simple pendant resting against the sternum or a bold bracelet encircling the wrist—can serve as a talisman of self-esteem. Select pieces that resonate with your personal story: perhaps a ring passed down through family that reminds you of generational resilience, or a necklace purchased to commemorate a milestone in self-discovery. Scarves offer versatility, draped around the shoulders to create a sense of enclosure, or tied at the waist to accentuate curves. Even everyday items like a colorful headband or a pair of distinctive earrings can become anchors of presence, catching your eye in the mirror and reinforcing the commitment to embodied confidence.

In partnered scenarios, props such as a silk ribbon or a small fan can facilitate playful exchanges that honor both personal boundaries and shared creativity. The act of tying a ribbon loosely around the wrist becomes a ritual of mutual trust, and the rising and falling of a fan can mirror the ebb and flow of emotional connection. These simple objects, handled with intention, become extensions of the body's language—tools that translate inner attunement into shared experience.

When fashion, movement, and accessories converge, they create a rich tapestry of erotic self-expression that transcends any single garment or gesture. The body emerges not as a problem to fix but as an ever-evolving canvas for self-celebration. Each morning, the act of choosing what to wear, how to move, and which tokens to carry becomes a reaffirmation of the journey toward self-love. Over time, these practices infuse daily life with a steady undercurrent of confidence, ensuring that the lessons of mirror work, dance improvisation, and art therapy ripple outward into every aspect of your being, inviting you to inhabit the world with authenticity and joy.

Chapter 6: Hormonal Health Across the Lifespan

6.1 Puberty to Young Adulthood

The journey from childhood into young adulthood is marked by profound transformations—biological, emotional, and social—that set the stage for a woman's lifelong relationship with her body and her sexuality. At the heart of this metamorphosis lies the hormonal orchestra that brings about menarche, shapes emerging patterns of desire, and guides early choices around contraception. Understanding these early years with clarity and compassion lays a foundation for consistent wellbeing, equipping young women with the knowledge and confidence to navigate their changing bodies, communicate their needs, and cultivate a healthy, empowered sense of self.

Long before the first menstrual flow arrives, subtle signals begin to ripple through a girl's body. Between the ages of eight and thirteen, the hypothalamus in the brain gradually increases its secretion of gonadotropin-releasing hormone, which in turn prompts the pituitary gland to release luteinizing hormone (LH) and follicle-stimulating hormone (FSH). These chemical messengers travel to the ovaries, where they encourage the maturation of ovarian follicles and the production of estrogen. The resulting rise in estrogen levels gives rise to thelarche—breast budding—followed by the appearance of pubic hair, growth spurts in height, and shifting body composition. For the young person experiencing these changes, the arrival of breasts and curves can spark excitement, pride, confusion, or even anxiety, depending on how openly these developments are discussed and supported within family, school, and peer circles.

Menarche—the first menstrual period—typically occurs approximately two years after breast budding, although the range can span from as early as eight or as late as sixteen. Preparing for this milestone involves more than supplying sanitary pads or tampons; it requires comprehensive body education that normalizes menstruation as a healthy, cyclical process. In practical terms, caregivers and educators can introduce the young girl to the anatomy of the reproductive system, explaining how the uterus builds and sheds its lining each month, and why this is a sign of fertility rather than a malfunction. Diagrams and anatomically correct models demystify internal structures, while guided discussions about common menstrual symptoms—cramps, mood fluctuations, breast tenderness—help normalize the ebb and flow of physical sensations.

Beyond factual information, facilitating healthy peer dialogue can transform what might feel like a secretive rite of passage into a shared, supportive experience. In schools or community groups, moderated circles allow girls to voice questions—"Is it normal to bleed for five days?" "What if I bleed through my clothes?"—and hear from older peers who recount their own first periods with candor and humor. Such exchanges build a sense of collective resilience, teaching younger girls that surprise spotting in gym class or heavy flows on the second day are bumps on a common road, not personal failures or sources of shame. In families where cultural taboos surround menstruation, fostering open conversation can be more challenging but all the more vital: exploring the historical roots of silence—whether religious beliefs or patriarchal norms—helps everyone see how stigmas arise and how they can be consciously dismantled.

As the reality of monthly bleeding settles in, the question of contraception often presses itself into young adulthood. Early contraceptive decisions represent more than a technical choice between pills or condoms; they invite a holistic evaluation of health, autonomy, and personal values. For many, the first step is a visit to a trusted healthcare provider—ideally someone who listens without judgment, clearly explains the mechanisms of different methods, and respects the young woman's right to confidentiality. A thorough discussion might cover hormonal options—combined estrogen-progestin pills, progestin-only "mini-pills," patches, and vaginal rings—as well as long-acting reversible contraceptives such as intrauterine devices (IUDs) or implants. Each method carries implications for menstrual regularity, side effects such as mood changes or weight fluctuations, and long-term fertility planning.

Non-hormonal alternatives also deserve careful consideration. Barrier methods—male or female condoms, diaphragms, and cervical caps—provide contraception without altering the body's own hormonal rhythms. Participants in peer support forums often attest to the sense of control they feel when they can physically handle and insert a diaphragm, trusting that no systemic hormones will shift their energy or mood. Natural family planning methods—tracking basal body temperature, cervical mucus changes, and menstrual cycle length—offer another route, though they require diligent daily monitoring and a clear understanding of fertile windows. Some young women combine methods, using condoms for both contraception and protection against sexually transmitted infections alongside a hormonal method chosen for its pattern of bleeding suppression or cycle regulation.

Holistic evaluation extends beyond the physical to embrace mental and emotional dimensions. When exploring hormonal contraceptives, it can be useful to keep a calendar journal for three to six months, documenting not only bleeding patterns but also mood, sleep quality, energy levels, and any emerging side effects. This process cultivates a nuanced understanding of one's own baseline, making it easier to discern whether headaches, irritability, or breast tenderness are linked to stress, diet, or the chosen contraceptive. Through patterns of observation, the young woman becomes her own best advocate, armed with concrete data when discussing potential adjustments—switching pill formulations, trying a lower-dose option, or exploring a non-hormonal alternative.

Amid these decisions, the emerging pulses of libido in late teens and early twenties often reflect the peak of hormonal vitality. Estrogen levels reach robust heights just prior to ovulation, priming the vaginal tissues for lubrication and the neural pathways for arousal. Testosterone, though present in lower quantities in women than in men, contributes to sexual desire, and its influence can feel particularly strong in the days leading up to and immediately following menarche, as well as in the years when ovarian reserve is at its maximum. Recognizing these cyclical surges offers a powerful tool for self-exploration: rather than labeling fluctuating desire as unpredictable or problematic, the young woman learns to see it as a conversation between her hormones and her embodied preferences.

Harnessing this hormonal peak involves experimenting with solo pleasure practices in a spirit of curiosity rather than performance. In the safety of a warm shower or the quietude of a penned-in journal session, she might track variation in self-stimulation techniques: a contrast between long, exploratory strokes and focused, rhythmic pulses; the impact of temperature play using warm water; or the subtler pleasure of mindful breathing and pelvic floor relaxation. Recording these experiments alongside cycle data illuminates which methods resonate most deeply during high-estrogen phases and which provide comfort or arousal when estrogen dips in the luteal or menstrual phases.

Such self-exploration serves dual purposes: it nurtures a positive relationship with bodily sensation and creates a detailed pleasure map that anticipates the rhythms of the menstrual cycle. When partnered intimacy arises, the young adult brings this inner knowledge to shared encounters, guiding a partner's touch or offering verbal feedback rooted in somatic awareness. The confidence gained in mapping personal pleasure becomes particularly potent when early contraceptive side effects—such as changes in lubrication or shifts in mood—challenge one's baseline. Equipped with the ability to self-soothe, to articulate what feels supportive or discordant, the young woman is less likely to internalize negative messages about her body's performance and more likely to advocate for adjustments—be it a contraceptive switch or a new approach to foreplay.

This interplay of cycle awareness, contraceptive choice, and libido exploration sets the stage for a lifetime of informed, empowered sexual health. The strategies learned in these formative years—menarche readiness through open education and peer support, holistic contraceptive evaluation with mindful self-tracking, and pleasure mapping aligned with hormonal fluctuations—form an integrated toolkit. As the young woman moves into her mid-twenties, these habits of observation and communication will anchor her through changes in partnership status, career demands, and evolving cultural narratives around sexuality. By viewing the teenage years not as a time to be endured but as a period rich with opportunity for self-discovery, she claims authorship of her own journey, learning to listen to the subtle wisdom of her hormones and to collaborate with them in crafting a consistent path of wellbeing and authentic intimacy.

6.2 Reproductive Years & Cyclical Awareness

Once past the early years of hormonal discovery, many women enter a period often referred to as their reproductive prime, brimming with cyclical patterns that can be harnessed as intuitive guides rather than sources of confusion. Central to this phase is mastering fertility awareness, a practice that transforms the seemingly unpredictable menstrual cycle into a valuable tool for understanding one's body and desire. Each morning, before rising from bed, you place a thermometer under your tongue or against your armpit, allowing a minute for an accurate basal body temperature reading. Over weeks, patterns emerge: a slight dip followed by a sustained rise signals ovulation, marking the days when estrogen surges and progesterone follows. Alongside temperature, you attend to cervical fluid—its shifting textures from scant and sticky after menstruation to creamy mid-cycle, then slippery and egg-white in the fertile window. You note these changes in a discreet journal or an app designed for cycle charting, juxtaposing them with mood observations: moments of grounded calm, bursts of energy, or days tinged with irritability.

This tapestry of data—temperature, fluid, mood—becomes your personal guidebook. Rather than seeing PMS as an unwelcome monthly guest, you recognize premenstrual symptoms as the body's way of signaling that estrogen is ebbing and progesterone is peaking. Perhaps a few days before menstruation you feel puffy, slightly melancholy, or prone to tension headaches. Armed with this knowledge, you adapt your self-care accordingly: choosing restorative yoga sequences over high-impact cardio, indulging in warm baths with magnesium salts, or planning evenings of gentle journaling instead of late-night socializing. Conversely, the pre-ovulatory rise in estrogen often brings clarity of thought, increased libido, and a sense of expansion. You might channel this energy into new creative projects, adventurous outings, or more spirited intimacy, knowing that your body is primed for higher arousal and emotional connection.

Embracing these hormonal rhythms shifts the relationship with one's own cycle from adversarial to collaborative. When partners are included in this awareness, intimacy deepens through mutual support. In weeks when you feel buoyant and social, your partner may arrange date nights or spontaneous gestures of affection. In the days when tenderness and slower pacing are needed, they might offer extra massages, cook comforting meals, or simply honor your need for space. Open dialogue about these fluctuations—saying "I feel most energized mid-cycle, and I'd love to plan something special"—invites shared responsibility for well-being, turning cyclical shifts into opportunities for connection rather than sources of misunderstanding.

The integration of cycle syncing into daily life extends beyond the bedroom. You might organize your work projects around phases of the cycle: tackling demanding tasks when cognitive focus peaks, and reserving planning and reflection for lower-energy days. Nutrition and exercise also adapt: lean proteins and complex carbohydrates can stabilize mood swings in the luteal phase, while light cardio and leafy greens support detoxification post-menstruation. By coordinating daily routines with the natural ebb and flow of hormones, you honor the body's ancient wisdom, reducing stress and fostering a sense of agency over your own biology.

Implementing cyclical awareness need not be overwhelming. Start simply by charting for one cycle, noting at least three parameters—temperature, cervical fluid quality, and a one-word mood descriptor. Reflect on these entries at month's end: what patterns did you notice? Did a surge in energy align with creative breakthroughs, or did premenstrual tension coincide with interpersonal friction? Use these insights to experiment in the next cycle: schedule a breathwork session two days before menstruation, or plan a weekend excursion three days before ovulation. As confidence grows, you may introduce additional tracking—such as libido ratings on a one-to-five scale or notes on sleep quality—but always ground the practice in curiosity rather than perfectionism.

Over time, reproductive awareness becomes woven into your sense of self. Rather than dreading irregularities, you learn to interpret them as signals warranting rest, medical consultation, or lifestyle tweaks. Missed ovulation may reveal signs of chronic stress or nutrient deficiencies; heavier flows might prompt a check for iron levels or thyroid function. In this way, cyclical awareness evolves into a holistic health practice, encompassing mindfulness, nutrition, movement, and emotional literacy. The dance of hormones, far from being an obstacle, transforms into a compass guiding you toward sustained vitality, deeper relationships, and a more attuned, resilient form of wellbeing.

6.3 Menopause, Perimenopause & Beyond

As the tapestry of reproductive years fades into the quieter plains of perimenopause and menopause, the body's hormonal landscape undergoes profound neuroendocrine shifts. Estrogen production by the ovaries wanes; the orchestrated rise and fall of estradiol and progesterone that once ruled the cycle gives way to irregular fluctuations, hot flashes, night sweats, and the gradual thinning of vaginal tissues. Understanding these changes reframes them not as a decline but as a natural evolution—an invitation to navigate later life intimacy with wisdom, creativity, and self-compassion.

Perimenopause, the transitional period before menopause, often begins in the mid-forties but can start earlier or later. During this phase, erratic estrogen levels may cause unpredictable menstrual cycles, making fertility awareness charting less reliable. Yet this unpredictability need not erode self-trust. By maintaining cycle logs, you can note missed periods, heavier bleeding, or extended spotting, all of which help you and your healthcare provider discern whether symptoms lie within normal perimenopausal variation or warrant further evaluation. Simultaneously, mood swings or irritability may emerge as estrogen dips, intersecting with life stressors—career transitions, aging parents, or evolving family roles. Recognizing these mood patterns as hormonally influenced rather than personal failings allows you to respond with targeted self-care: herbal adaptogens such as black cohosh or chasteberry may bring relief, while integrative practices like acupuncture or mindfulness meditation soothe the nervous system's reactivity.

Menopause itself is diagnosed after twelve consecutive months without menstruation. At this juncture, estrogen levels settle at a new baseline, and the risk of osteoporosis and cardiovascular issues rises due to the protective effects of estrogen receding. You may also notice decreased natural lubrication, making intercourse less comfortable. Vaginal tissues thin and lose elasticity, a process called atrophy, which can be addressed through pelvic floor exercises and the use of water-based lubricants or vaginal moisturizers. Over-the-counter options provide immediate comfort, while prescription treatments, such as low-dose vaginal estrogen creams or rings, deliver localized hormone support without significantly affecting systemic levels. Discussing these approaches openly with a healthcare provider ensures that you choose interventions aligned with your overall health profile and personal preferences.

For those seeking broader hormonal balance, the decision between bioidentical and synthetic hormone replacement therapy (HRT) can feel weighty. Bioidentical hormones are formulated to chemically match the body's own estrogen and progesterone molecules. Proponents argue that this molecular fidelity reduces side effects and offers a more natural transition. However, the research remains mixed, and compounded bioidentical creams or pills prescribed through certain pharmacies may lack the rigorous testing standards of pharmaceutical products. Synthetic HRT, regulated and tested through large clinical trials, provides well-studied formulations—such as conjugated equine estrogens or medroxyprogesterone—that have documented benefits and risks. Conversations with a knowledgeable clinician should explore factors such as personal and family history of breast cancer or cardiovascular disease, the severity of menopausal symptoms, and one's priorities for quality of life. Whether bioidentical or synthetic, HRT is never a one-size-fits-all solution; the optimal regimen is highly individual, requiring careful monitoring and periodic reassessment.

Yet even without systemic HRT, many women discover what is sometimes called a "second blooming" in later life—an era marked by newfound freedom, creative energy, and a deeper sense of self that blossoms once the unpredictability of monthly cycles recedes. Freed from the demands of contraception and cyclical planning, you may explore forms of intimacy that previously felt out of reach. Morning routines that once revolved around menstrual products now include leisurely stretches or dance flows that celebrate the body's resilience. Intimate rituals—such as candlelit baths with aromatic oils, gentle pelvic floor massage, or shared storytelling with a partner—take on new significance, honoring the wisdom accrued over decades of experience.

Community also plays a transformative role in this phase. Joining peer groups geared toward perimenopausal or menopausal women fosters a sense of solidarity and normalizes conversations about hot flashes, sleep disturbances, and shifting desire. Within these circles, members exchange practical tips—cooling scarves, mindfulness apps for night sweats, or favorite music playlists that lift the spirit during momentary waves of anxiety. They also celebrate one another's "second blooms": an artist finding inspiration for a new medium, a couple rediscovering playful intimacy, or a career pivot that aligns more deeply with personal purpose.

Ultimately, the passage through menopause and beyond invites a redefinition of sexuality and self-care, one that embraces altered hormones not as a loss but as a recalibration. With a compassionate understanding of neuroendocrine changes, thoughtful choices around hormone therapy, and an openness to creative reinvention, you can cultivate an empowered, joyous chapter of life. Here, the body's wisdom shines brightest, its voice unencumbered by the tumult of monthly cycles, offering an opportunity for intimate connection that is at once serene, authentic, and deeply enlivened by the richness of lived experience.

Chapter 7: Holistic Practices for Sexual Wellbeing

7.1 Integrative Movement: Yoga, Dance & Pilates

For countless women, the pursuit of sexual wellbeing has too often meant a narrow focus on symptom management—medications to address low libido, lubricants for discomfort, or counseling only when difficulties become acute. Yet a growing body of evidence suggests that integrative movement modalities—practices rooted in ancient traditions and modern exercise science alike—can offer a deeply supportive path to vitality, resilience, and pleasure. Women who embrace these holistic approaches report significantly fewer symptoms of sexual dysfunction than those who rely exclusively on pharmaceuticals. In this section, we explore three pillars of integrative movement—yoga, dance, and Pilates—each of which can be adapted to cultivate pelvic floor tone, deepen mind–body connection, and awaken the body's natural capacity for sensation and confidence.

Yoga, with its millennia-old lineage, provides a rich vocabulary of postures and breathwork techniques that can be tailored specifically to the needs of the pelvic floor and surrounding musculature. While many are familiar with general hatha or vinyasa sequences, a pelvic-floor–focused yoga practice zeroes in on what yogis call the mula bandha, or root lock—a subtle lift and engagement of the muscles at the base of the torso. To begin, practitioners are guided into a comfortable seated position, perhaps on a folded blanket or bolster, with the spine tall and the sit bones grounded. The initial invitation is to draw awareness inward, placing hands gently over the lower belly and pelvic area to sense the natural expansion and contraction of breath. With each inhale, the breath fills the lower belly, creating a gentle outward pressure. As the exhale unfolds, the mula bandha engages: the muscles of the pelvic floor lift slightly, pulling upward toward the navel. This movement can be likened to a soft "zippering" sensation, as though the base of the torso is being drawn toward the heart.

Early sessions focus on refining that internal cue—coordinating breath with gentle, rhythmic contractions—to establish a neural pathway between mind and muscle. The tempo is slow, perhaps five seconds of lift on the exhale, followed by five seconds of release on the inhale. Over time, women report greater ease in isolating the pelvic floor, noticing subtle shifts that once went undetected. Building on this foundation, the practice may introduce supported bridge poses, with the feet hip-distance apart and the shoulders and head resting on the mat. As the hips lift, the practitioner continues to engage mula bandha, creating stability through the pelvis and lower back. This combination of lift and breath encourages not only muscular tone but also proprioceptive awareness—the ability to feel where the body is in space, a crucial component of comfortable, pleasurable movement.

Flowing between postures, the sequence might incorporate dynamic variations such as supported goddess pose, legs bent and open wide, toes turned outward, as the breath guides the torso into gentle side bends. With palms pressed together at the heart or extended overhead, the practitioner feels the pelvic floor respond to shifts in gravity and hip alignment. Each movement becomes an experiment in coordination: How does the lift of mula bandha change when the hips move laterally? What subtle adjustments in foot placement facilitate a more stable foundation? This investigative stance, free from the pressure to achieve a perfect shape, fosters a spirit of curiosity and self-compassion—qualities that enrich sexual wellbeing by dispelling shame and inviting exploration.

Dance, in its many forms, offers another avenue for integrative movement, one that celebrates the body's expressive potential and awakens hip mobility in particular. Sensual dance flows—sophisticated sequences that blend elements of contemporary dance, floorwork, and improvisation—give women permission to inhabit their bodies with confidence, texture, and rhythm. A typical class might begin with a grounding exercise: standing in a wide second position with knees softly bent, the dancer rocks from side to side, feeling the weight transfer from one leg to the other. As this gentle sway tunes the nervous system to receptivity, the instructor introduces a series of hip isolations—tiny circles, tilts, and figure-eights—that warm up the sacroiliac joints and deepen awareness of the pelvic basin.

Rather than mechanical drills, these hip mobilizations are woven into larger, flowing patterns. One might undulate the torso in a wave-like motion, the sequence beginning at the crown of the head, cascading through shoulders, rib cage, and culminating in a soft, circular sweep of the hips. Music with a languid, pulsing beat supports the tempo, encouraging the dancer to find her own timing within the flow. As sequences progress, the choreography may incorporate shifts in level—bending into a low squat with thighs pressing outward, then rising to a full lengthening of the spine—always with attention to the pelvis's subtle tilts and rotations. Over weeks of practice, participants often report increased hip flexibility, reduced stiffness in the lower back, and a heightened body-mind connection that translates into more fluid movement both on and off the dance floor.

Beyond structured steps, improvisation plays a central role in dance flows for sexual wellbeing. In guided improvisations, the instructor might prompt participants to explore the question "What does confidence feel like in my body?" inviting each woman to respond with three movements that embody her own sense of authority and radiance. One person's answer might be a firm stomping of the feet; another's a delicate, spiraling extension of the arm. By honoring each unique expression, the practice reinforces the principle that there is no single "correct" way to move—or to be. When bodies learn to move with agency, trust, and playful curiosity, the benefits extend beyond flexibility to include an unspoken permission to inhabit one's own skin without apology.

Pilates, with its roots in early twentieth-century rehabilitation and physical fitness, offers a complementary toolkit for fortifying the deep core muscles that underlie both posture and sexual function. While casual observers may associate Pilates solely with long, lean limbs and mat exercises, a pelvic-floor–informed Pilates regimen highlights the transverse abdominis—a corset-like layer of muscle that wraps around the torso—and its synergy with the pelvic floor. Coursework often begins with supine abdominal engagement: lying on the back with knees bent and feet flat on the floor, practitioners draw the navel gently toward the spine, activating the transverse abdominis without gripping the rectus abdominis or straining the neck. With the breath anchored into the lower belly, they then coordinate a subtle engagement of the pelvic floor, integrating it seamlessly with the core contraction.

Bridging exercises in Pilates expand this connection. As the hips lift into a bridge, the core remains drawn inward, preventing the lower back from overarching, while the pelvic floor sustains a light lift. Holding the bridge position for several breaths strengthens the posterior chain—glutes and hamstrings—while the simultaneous engagement of front and bottom core supports pelvic stability. For those ready to advance, Pilates apparatus such as the Reformer or the Cadillac offers variable resistance to challenge coordination. Springs pull the carriage away from the footbar, requiring a precise balance of core and pelvic-floor engagement to maintain control as the legs extend. Each repetition reinforces the neural pathway that links breath, core activation, and pelvic floor lift—a triad that supports both everyday posture and the physiological processes underlying optimal sexual function.

In addition to strengthening, Pilates emphasizes controlled movement quality and mind–body focus. Slow, deliberate exercises—leg circles with hips held steady, side-lying lifts with rotation—invite the practitioner to notice the subtleties of muscle recruitment. Does the outer hip begin to—buttock—to compensate for insufficient transverse abdominis activation? Does the breath unconsciously shift to the upper chest? By attending to these nuances, women develop a refined proprioception that carries over into moments of intimacy: they become adept at sensing and modulating tension, discovering how a slight adjustment in pelvic tilt can either open or close pathways of sensation.

Integrating yoga, dance, and Pilates into a cohesive movement practice need not require lengthy daily sessions or professional studios. Even short, focused routines performed three times a week can yield noticeable improvements in pelvic stability, hip flexibility, and core strength—all of which contribute to greater comfort, confidence, and ease of movement in intimate contexts. A typical micro-practice might begin with a brief mula bandha sequence in seated meditation, followed by five minutes of hip-opening dance improvisation accompanied by favorite music, concluding with a trio of Pilates-inspired bridges or leg-lowering exercises on the mat. Over time, these bite-sized sessions accumulate into significant gains: tension patterns in the pelvis dissolve, posture improves, and a sense of muscular empowerment takes root.

Beyond the physical benefits, integrative movement practices cultivate an attitudinal shift toward the body: from object of critique to partner in exploration. The textures of muscle engagement, the rhythms of breathed movement, and the creative play of dance all remind practitioners that the body is inherently intelligent and responsive. When posture, flexibility, and strength grow in tandem with mindfulness and curiosity, women discover an embodied assurance that permeates every aspect of life— including the realm of intimacy. In this sense, yoga, dance, and Pilates do more than tone muscles; they weave a tapestry of connection between mind, body, and heart, supporting a sexual wellbeing that is as robust as it is nuanced. As you continue on your journey, let these integrative movement practices serve not as chores to check off, but as invitations to come home to your body's vibrant aliveness—one breath, one step, one lifted pelvic floor at a time.

7.2 Breathwork, Meditation & Nervous System Regulation

The intricate dance between breath, mind, and body holds untapped potential for cultivating a nervous system receptive to pleasure and intimacy. In our fast-paced world, the sympathetic "fight-or-flight" state often predominates, leaving little room for the parasympathetic response that underlies relaxation, connection, and desire. Breathwork and meditation practices offer accessible yet profound methods for shifting off the sympathetic highway and into the parasympathetic back roads, where the vagus nerve can sing its soothing song and the body rediscovers its capacity for ease and openness.

One of the most direct ways to engage the parasympathetic system is through coherent breathing, a simple technique in which inhales and exhales are matched in length and paced at approximately five seconds each. To begin, find a comfortable seated position—ideally upright yet relaxed, with hands resting gently on the thighs and eyes softly closed. On an inhale that lasts silently to the count of five, feel the breath move first into the belly, then expand the ribs, and finally lift the chest. Pause briefly at the top of the inhale, then release the breath over a five-count exhale, sensing the abdomen draw back toward the spine, the ribs gently contract, and the chest return to its resting position. As you continue this rhythm—inhale for five, exhale for five—the heart rate slows, blood pressure dips, and the vagal tone increases, effectively flipping the switch from anxiety toward calm. With regular practice, even a few minutes of coherent breathing can reduce cortisol levels and prime the nervous system for experiences of connection and pleasure.

Once coherent breathing has re-established a baseline of calm, guided imagery can further deepen the shift into parasympathetic responsiveness. Although the word "erotic" may evoke images of explicit content, erotic imagery in this context refers to scenes and sensations that gently beckon the body into relaxation and arousal through vivid, multisensory storytelling. Imagine, for example, a guided visualization in which you find yourself walking barefoot along a sun-warmed shoreline at dusk. You feel the grain of sand beneath your soles, the gentle lapping of water against your ankles, and a warm breeze that brushes across your skin like a soft caress. As you move through the scene, the guide's voice encourages you to notice the subtle warmth at the base of the spine, to allow your belly to soften and your breath to deepen, to sense an opening in the chest that invites both confidence and vulnerability. By layering tactile, auditory, and emotional elements, these visualizations prime the parasympathetic system in a way that mirrors the sensations of intimacy, without requiring a partner or physical proximity.

The choice of meditation technique further influences how effectively the mind–body connection supports sexual wellbeing. Transcendental Meditation (TM), for instance, employs the repetition of a personal mantra given by a certified instructor. Practitioners typically sit comfortably with eyes closed, silently repeating the mantra for twenty minutes, twice a day. The effortless, mantra-based focus bypasses discursive thought and fosters a deep, restful state akin to the restorative phase of sleep. Studies have shown that TM practitioners exhibit enhanced vagal tone, reduced anxiety, and improved overall wellbeing—factors that indirectly benefit sexual function by reducing the cognitive chatter and stress that often inhibit desire.

In contrast, mindfulness meditation cultivates moment-to-moment awareness without judgment, often by focusing on the breath or bodily sensations. A simple mindfulness practice might begin by anchoring attention on the flow of each inhale and exhale, noticing the rise and fall of the abdomen and the passage of air through the nostrils. When thoughts intrude—plans for tomorrow, worries about performance—the practitioner gently acknowledges them as passing clouds and returns focus to the breath. Over time, this practice strengthens the prefrontal cortex's capacity to regulate the amygdala's reactivity, diminishing the freeze-or-flee response and allowing the subtle signals of arousal and comfort to surface more easily.

Choosing between transcendental and mindfulness meditation depends on personal preference and lifestyle. TM's scripted structure can be appealing for those who appreciate a clearly defined process and who have the resources to learn from a certified teacher. Its barrier to entry may feel higher, but the deep states of rest it produces can yield rapid benefits in stress reduction. Mindfulness, on the other hand, offers greater flexibility: minutes-long practices can be woven into daily routines without formal instruction, and a myriad of free resources—apps, online videos, group classes—support beginners. Some women find a blended approach most effective: engaging in TM to cultivate deep respite and practicing mindfulness in moments of daily stress or prior to intimacy to maintain presence and attunement.

Ultimately, breathwork and meditation serve as bridges into the parasympathetic domain, where connection, sensation, and pleasure can flourish. By establishing coherent breathing as a foundational habit, employing guided visualizations to evoke the gentle thrill of intimacy, and selecting a meditation style that resonates, women can retrain their nervous systems. Over weeks and months, these practices carve new neural pathways that favor calm and openness, transforming the mind–body relationship from one of tension and distraction into one of receptive aliveness. As a result, both solo and partnered experiences become richer, more fulfilling encounters with the body's inherent capacity for delight and connection.

7.3 Nutritional, Herbal & Supplement Support

Just as movement and breathwork sculpt the body's physical and neurological landscape, nutrition and targeted supplementation lay the chemical foundation for balanced hormones, robust energy, and optimal circulation—key ingredients in a vibrant sexual life. By incorporating adaptogens, essential micronutrients, and anti-inflammatory dietary patterns, women can address root causes of low libido, fatigue, and discomfort, creating a nutrient environment that supports both physical health and sensual vitality.

Adaptogenic herbs have surged in popularity for their reputed ability to modulate the body's stress response, offering balanced support to the adrenal and endocrine systems. Ashwagandha, a staple of Ayurvedic medicine, exemplifies this category. When taken consistently—as a standardized root extract in capsule form or blended into warm milk—ashwagandha has been shown in clinical trials to reduce cortisol levels, improve sleep quality, and enhance overall sense of wellbeing. These effects indirectly benefit sexual desire by easing the chronic activation of the stress response that suppresses reproductive hormones. Unique to ashwagandha is its potential to impact libido directly: small studies indicate improved sexual satisfaction and lubrication in women experiencing stress-related low desire.

Maca root, cultivated for centuries in the high Andes, provides another adaptogenic profile, often touted for its energizing properties. Available as a flour-like powder, maca can be stirred into smoothies, oatmeal, or warm beverages, providing a mild nutty flavor. Research suggests that maca may support balanced estrogen levels and enhance sexual function, possibly through its content of bioactive compounds such as macamides and macaenes. Women experimenting with maca often report subtle improvements in stamina, mood, and spontaneous desire, particularly when used regularly over a two- to three-month period.

Rhodiola rosea, indigenous to Arctic regions, rounds out the trio of popular adaptogens. Known for its capacity to bolster mental resilience and reduce fatigue, rhodiola works in part by supporting the availability of neurotransmitters such as serotonin and dopamine—molecules integral to both mood regulation and the experience of pleasure. For women who find that stress and low energy dampen their sexual interest, rhodiola offers a targeted approach to invigorating the nervous system without the jittery side effects of stimulants.

Complementing adaptogens, certain micronutrients serve as cofactors in hormone synthesis and neuromodulation. Zinc, often discussed in the context of men's health, plays a crucial role in women's reproductive function as well. It participates in the regulation of ovarian hormones and the maintenance of tissue integrity, including vaginal mucosa. Magnesium, a mineral lost readily through stress and sweat, supports the body's relaxation response by helping to regulate calcium channels in muscle and nerve cells. It also contributes to healthy sleep patterns—an essential precondition for balanced desire. B-vitamins, particularly B6 and B12, aid in the metabolism of amino acids that serve as precursors for dopamine and serotonin, neurotransmitters that influence both mood and sexual arousal. By ensuring adequate intake of these micronutrients—whether through a varied diet or a high-quality, gender-specific multivitamin—women lay the groundwork for hormonal harmony and energy stability.

Beyond individual herbs and nutrients, adopting an anti-inflammatory dietary pattern can address pelvic discomfort, improve circulation, and reduce systemic inflammation that may underlie conditions such as endometriosis or interstitial cystitis. An anti-inflammatory meal plan emphasizes whole, minimally processed foods: colorful vegetables, fatty fish rich in omega-3s, nuts and seeds, whole grains, and antioxidant-rich fruits such as berries. Herbs and spices—turmeric with its curcumin compound, ginger, garlic, and fresh leafy greens—provide additional anti-inflammatory phytochemicals. In practice, a day on such a diet might begin with a bowl of steel-cut oats topped with mixed berries, chia seeds, and a dash of cinnamon; a midday plate balancing wild salmon over a bed of quinoa and roasted Brussels sprouts; and an evening stir-fry of tofu, kale, bell peppers, and turmeric, served with a side of brown rice. Snacks of raw nuts or a green smoothie featuring spinach, banana, and a scoop of maca powder sustain energy without provoking blood sugar spikes.

To further personalize the anti-inflammatory approach, women may explore elimination diets—temporarily removing common irritants such as gluten, dairy, soy, or refined sugars and then reintroducing them one by one to gauge individual tolerance. A four-week pilot can reveal whether certain foods exacerbate pelvic pain, mood lability, or bloating, enabling targeted adjustments rather than broad dietary restriction. Keeping a simple food-mood-symptom log—detailing what was eaten, how one felt emotionally, and any physical discomfort—guides iteration and fine-tuning.

Finally, pairing dietary shifts with mindful eating practices enhances both nutrient absorption and the embodied experience of food. Sitting down without screens, chewing slowly, and savouring flavours allows the parasympathetic system to engage during meals, optimizing digestive function and fostering a deeper connection to the body's signals of satisfaction. As digestion improves, so too do energy levels and hormonal balance—factors that ripple outward into greater interest in intimacy and improved comfort in the pelvic region.

Together, these nutritional, herbal, and supplement strategies forge a biochemical landscape in which sexual wellbeing can flourish. By choosing adaptogens that soothe the stress response, ensuring key micronutrients for hormone production, and embracing anti-inflammatory foods that support circulation and reduce discomfort, women equip themselves with a comprehensive toolkit for sustaining desire, comfort, and vitality. When combined with integrative movement and breath-based practices, this holistic framework addresses the body's needs at every level—mind, body, and spirit—creating a resilient foundation for enduring sexual health and joy.

Chapter 8: Integrating Sexuality with Overall Wellness

8.1 Sexual Fitness: Strength, Endurance & Flexibility

When we think of exercise, spinning classes or weightlifting sessions often come to mind, while the role of sexual activity in our overall fitness tends to be overlooked. Yet, an intimate encounter can burn between one hundred and three hundred calories, elevate heart rate, and recruit muscle groups from head to toe, delivering benefits akin to more conventional workouts. Recognizing sexuality as a legitimate component of one's fitness routine opens new pathways to health: by deliberately cultivating strength, endurance, and flexibility in ways that serve both everyday life and intimate moments, women lay a foundation for vitality that extends far beyond the bedroom.

At the heart of intimate fitness lies pelvic floor conditioning, most commonly known as Kegel exercises. These movements target the sling of muscles that supports the bladder, uterus, and bowel, and that plays a key role in sexual response by modulating sensation and control. A basic Kegel begins with finding the muscles: as if stopping the flow of urine or holding in gas, one lifts and squeezes the pelvic floor. Initially, simple holds of three to five seconds—followed by equal-length releases—suffice to build awareness. Practitioners often sit on a firm chair or lie supine with knees bent, resting a hand on the lower abdomen to ensure that only pelvic floor muscles, not the glutes or thighs, are engaged. Sensations may be subtle at first; with patience, the nervous system learns to isolate and activate those deep muscles.

As proficiency grows, the routine evolves into progressive Kegel sequences. Instead of static holds, pulses—quick lifts and releases at a one-second rhythm—introduce an endurance component. After a warm-up of ten steady holds, a set of twenty pulses challenges the muscle fibers in a different way, enhancing blood flow and neuromuscular coordination. Over weeks, the holds lengthen to ten or even fifteen seconds, with equal rest periods between. To elevate resistance, one can employ specialized pelvic-floor bands or small silicone pessary-like cones: inserting the device and lifting against its gentle weight encourages stronger contractions. Some women integrate biofeedback tools—small sensors that translate pelvic floor engagement into visual or auditory signals—further refining control. Through these progressions, the pelvic floor transforms from an unnoticed foundation into an actively engaged network, improving bladder support, spinal stability, and the subtle dance of arousal and release that underpins satisfying intimacy.

While solo work on the mat strengthens the core, partnering up for body-weight exercises introduces a playful, mutual dimension to strength-building. In a simple seated-back-to-back press, partners sit on the floor with knees bent and press their shoulder blades together to create resistance while inhaling and exhaling in synchrony. This press not only engages the erector spinae muscles but also invites attunement to each other's breath patterns. Another move involves one person in a high plank while the other lightly places hands on their lower back, providing subtle weight that increases the plank's challenge. As the person in plank holds the position, the partner can shift their hands gently, encouraging micro-adjustments that enhance core stability and proprioception. Swap roles after thirty seconds or one minute, ensuring both build endurance.

Squats add a dynamic element: facing each other, partners hold forearms and descend together into a squat, synchronizing breath and movement. The shared support helps maintain proper form—hips back, knees tracking over toes—and transforms a routine set of repetitions into a co-created exercise, reinforcing trust and playful connection. For a more adventurous variation, one partner holds a side plank while the other performs a dip under their extended legs, then reverses. This move calls upon lateral core strength and hip flexor engagement in both individuals, all within a context of cooperative movement that heightens mutual awareness.

Beyond strength and endurance, flexibility underpins fluid, comfortable movement in both daily life and intimate encounters. Tight hips and lower backs are especially common among women who work long hours seated or who habitually adopt postures that favor one side of the body. Addressing these imbalances begins with a mindful sequence of stretches performed with steady, diaphragmatic breathing. A low lunge—stepping the right foot forward and lowering the left knee to the mat—releases tension in the left hip flexor and quadriceps. As the breath deepens, the pelvis can tilt posteriorly, intensifying the stretch while the torso remains tall. After thirty to sixty seconds, switching sides ensures symmetrical mobility.

Moving into a more restorative stretch, the figure-four position—lying supine with the right ankle crossing the left thigh just above the knee—opens the right hip. Gently drawing the left thigh toward the chest, the practitioner feels a pronounced release through the gluteus medius and piriformis muscles. Holding for a minute or two on each side, this drill soothes common sources of lower back discomfort and counterbalances the demands of Kegel strengthening.

The lower back itself benefits from gentle rotation drills. Seated or supine, turning the knees to the side with the shoulders remaining square creates a soft spinal twist, inviting each vertebra to articulate. Interspersed with cat-cow sequences— moving the spine between arch and rounding while on hands and knees—these movements lubricate the intervertebral joints and reduce stiffness that can inhibit comfortable movement. Shoulders, often rounded forward in modern posture, require their own attention. Anchoring a resistance band or simply grasping a towel behind the back and lifting allows a gentle stretch across the chest and anterior shoulders. Alternatively, standing in a doorway and placing forearms on the frame at shoulder height, the chest can sink forward, opening the pectoral muscles and allowing the shoulder blades to glide toward the spine.

Together, these strength, endurance, and flexibility practices compose an integrated regimen that supports sexual wellbeing at multiple levels. The act of engaging pelvic floor muscles cultivates strength and control where it matters most, while partner-based exercises transform routine strength work into shared experiences that build trust and attunement. Flexibility drills dissolve the habitual tension that can block comfortable movement, restoring resilience and grace. When woven into a weekly routine—perhaps two days of Kegel progressions, two days of partner strength work, and daily flexibility sequences— this holistic approach fosters a body that is strong yet supple, energized yet relaxed.

Most importantly, the mindset surrounding these practices unleashes their full power. Approaching each movement with curiosity and gratitude—attuning to subtle shifts, valuing incremental improvements, and celebrating the body's capacity for adaptation—reframes exercise from a task to be endured into an invitation to connect more deeply with one's own physical presence. In this spirit, sexual fitness emerges not as a separate silo of activity but as an integral thread woven through the fabric of everyday life, enhancing posture, easing tension, supporting mental clarity, and nourishing the energetic vitality that fuels both personal wellbeing and intimate connection. By embracing strength, endurance, and flexibility through the lens of holistic movement, women gain not only healthier bodies but also a richer relationship with their own aliveness—an outcome that resonates far beyond any single workout or encounter.

8.2 Sleep, Recovery & Libido Optimization

Sleep is often the unsung hero of sexual health. The architecture of a full night's rest—cycling through stages of light sleep, deep slow-wave sleep, and the vivid dreaming of rapid eye movement (REM)—plays a pivotal role in regulating the hormones that underlie desire. During REM sleep, the brain's limbic system, which governs emotion and arousal, becomes especially active. It is in this stage that levels of testosterone and estrogen are balanced, mood is regulated, and the brain consolidates memories, including those tied to intimacy and connection. When REM sleep is disrupted—whether by late-night screen time, stress-induced awakenings, or fragmented breathing—those hormonal fluctuations are thrown off course. Testosterone production in the evening and early morning hours can fall, leading to diminished libido, while estrogen imbalances may contribute to mood swings and vaginal dryness. Over time, a chronic deficit in REM sleep can erode sexual confidence, leaving a sense of fatigue that extends beyond physical tiredness into emotional detachment.

Cultivating an evening ritual can anchor the day's end and prepare the mind–body system for restorative sleep. Such a ritual begins by dimming electronic screens at least an hour before bedtime to reduce blue-light exposure, which suppresses the natural release of melatonin. In the soft glow of a bedside lamp or candlelight, one might turn to journaling, gently unloading the day's worries onto paper. By writing freely—perhaps noting three moments of gratitude, or simply listing tasks for tomorrow—mental clutter is externalized, reducing the likelihood of midnight rumination. Incorporating aromatherapy into this practice intensifies the soothing effect. A few drops of lavender or chamomile essential oil diffused in the bedroom, or gently applied to pulse points, can lower heart rate and quiet racing thoughts. As the journal closes, a brief sequence of light movement—slow stretches that hug the lower back, gentle side bends that massage the ribs, and a handful of relaxation breaths—signals to the nervous system that exertion is complete and restoration can begin. With the body warm, the mind decluttered, and the senses calmed, descending into deep sleep becomes a rhythmic, almost ritualistic act of self-care.

Napping, too, can serve as a strategic tool for hormonal reset and mood enhancement, especially for women juggling busy schedules or struggling to secure uninterrupted nighttime rest. Short "desire naps" of twenty to thirty minutes, ideally taken in the early afternoon, can boost testosterone levels by giving the adrenal glands a brief respite. The key is timing: a nap longer than forty minutes risks drifting into deep slow-wave sleep, which can leave one groggy upon waking, whereas a micro-nap of ten to fifteen minutes may not provide enough restorative benefit. By setting an alarm and finding a comfortable, dimly lit space—perhaps on a recliner or cushioned floor mat—women can afford themselves a mini-vacation from stress hormones and mental chatter. Emerging from a desire nap often brings a gentle freshness of mind, a subtle uplift in mood, and a renewed capacity to feel connected to one's body. When integrated thoughtfully into the weekly routine, these brief periods of recovery become potent allies in sustaining libido and emotional well-being.

8.3 Mental Health Synergies: Therapy, Coaching & Community

Sexual wellbeing is not solely a matter of biology; it unfolds within the rich terrain of our thoughts, emotions, and relationships. For many women, unresolved anxieties, ingrained negative beliefs about intimacy, or past traumas can overshadow even the best self-care practices. Integrated sex therapy models offer a bridge between cognitive insight and embodied experience, often combining elements of cognitive-behavioral therapy (CBT) with sensate focus techniques originally developed by masters in the field of sexology. In a typical integrated session, the therapist guides the client in identifying unhelpful thought patterns—such as catastrophizing ("If I don't perform perfectly, my partner will leave me") or all-or-nothing beliefs ("I should always feel desire, or something is wrong"). Through CBT exercises, these thoughts are gently challenged and reframed into more realistic, compassionate alternatives. Simultaneously, sensate focus practice invites women and, if applicable, their partners to engage in a sequence of non-goal-oriented touch exercises. Beginning with simple hand-holding or caressing of the arms, the exercises progress at a pace set by the client's comfort, allowing the nervous system to rebuild trust in the body's capacity for pleasurable sensation. Over time, the reflective work of CBT and the reparative power of sensate focus converge, dissolving performance anxiety and enabling a more relaxed, present-moment engagement with intimacy.

Beyond one-on-one therapy, many women find that group coaching pods provide an energizing synergy of peer accountability and shared learning. These small cohorts—often facilitated by trained coaches specializing in sexual confidence—meet regularly to explore themes such as boundary-setting, communication skills, and pleasure mapping. Within the safety of the pod, members share personal insights, celebrate one another's breakthroughs, and offer encouragement when challenges arise. This model leverages the power of collective momentum: witnessing a peer successfully negotiate a difficult conversation with a partner can serve as a catalyst for one's own courage; celebrating someone else's rediscovery of desire can normalize the fluctuations inherent in every woman's sexual journey. Unlike large support groups where sharing can feel impersonal, coaching pods maintain intimacy of scale—typically six to eight women—ensuring that each voice is heard, each victory acknowledged. The structured nature of coaching, with clear learning objectives and practical takeaways, also ensures that insights translate into concrete, actionable steps rather than remaining abstract aspirations.

When exploring group versus individual formats, the question often arises: should one turn to online or in-person support? The answer depends on personal preference, availability, and the nature of one's challenges. In-person networks, whether therapy groups or workshops, offer the richness of physical co-presence: the warmth of a shared room, nonverbal cues that deepen empathy, and informal interactions before or after sessions that can spark new connections. They can be particularly potent for those who value real-time feedback and the accountability that comes from showing up face-to-face. But online platforms bring their own strengths: they expand access to specialized expertise beyond one's geographic area, allow participation at flexible times, and often provide asynchronous discussion boards where members can post reflections at any moment. Privacy settings and anonymous profiles can foster candid sharing for those who feel reticent in public forums. In choosing a platform, it is crucial to assess whether the community upholds evidence-based practices—does the facilitator adhere to professional guidelines? Are resources grounded in peer-reviewed research? Is there a clear code of confidentiality and respect?

Regardless of format, the effectiveness of mental health synergies hinges on creating spaces that prioritize safety, inclusivity, and a commitment to ongoing growth. Whether in the sanctuary of a therapist's office, the structured environment of a coaching pod, or the boundless reach of an online forum, women find that aligning therapeutic insight with community support ignites transformations that neither modality could achieve alone. As thoughts become kinder, bodies more trusting, and connections more authentic, the journey toward sexual wellbeing unfolds not as a solitary quest but as a shared adventure, woven into the larger tapestry of mental health, personal empowerment, and collective flourishing.

Chapter 9: Sexual Empowerment & Agency

9.1 Overcoming Shame & Guilt

For many women, the journey toward sexual empowerment begins not in acts of exploration but in the long, often invisible struggle against shame and guilt. These emotions, woven through family teachings, cultural norms, and personal experiences, can create an almost imperceptible barrier to claiming agency over one's own body. Yet research shows that women who feel confident in setting their own boundaries, voicing their desires, and making informed choices are three times more likely to pursue and achieve satisfying relationships. Addressing shame and guilt, therefore, becomes a foundational act of reclaiming power—an act that unshackles the body, mind, and heart from the chains of judgment and opens the way to authentic expression.

At the core of shame resilience work, as articulated by scholar Brené Brown, lies a three-step process: naming, witnessing, and reaching out. Naming is the act of calling shame by its name, of recognizing the texture of the emotion when it arises. Shame can feel like a tightening in the throat, a sinking in the chest, or a prickly flush of heat in the face. It may appear whenever a thought crosses your mind—"I shouldn't feel this way," "I'm too much," "I'm not enough"—and drives you to hide or withdraw. In a moment of shame resilience, you pause and say to yourself: "This is shame. I see you." With naming, the experience shifts from an indefinable, overwhelming wave to a recognizable visitor, one that can be observed rather than mistaken for the whole of your being.

Witnessing follows naturally. Instead of pushing shame away or getting lost in its narrative, you attend to its presence with compassionate curiosity. Imagine sitting beside shame like a concerned friend: "I notice you're here. You're telling me that I did something wrong, that I'm flawed." In that stance, shame becomes something that happens to you, not something you are. Breathing deeply, you allow the emotion to be present without trying to fix, suppress, or indulge it. Witnessing creates a space of grace in which shame's voice can be heard but does not dominate the conversation. Over time, this practice rewires the neural pathways that once equated shame with self-erasure, replacing them with circuits of self-inquiry and understanding.

Reaching out constitutes the final, and perhaps most transformative, element of shame resilience. Shame thrives on secrecy and isolation; when we keep our experiences buried, shame festers. But sharing our stories of vulnerability—whether with a trusted friend, a therapist, or a support group—dilutes shame's power. By saying, "I felt guilty about my own desire," or "I was ashamed of my body's responses," we discover that others have felt similarly. Recognition, empathy, and solidarity flow through these conversations, cultivating connection and empathy. Each time we speak shame's truths out loud, we claim a little more agency and remind ourselves that we are not alone in our humanity.

Parallel to this shame resilience framework, inner-child dialogues offer a complementary path toward healing learned taboos. From our earliest years, we internalize messages—sometimes explicit, sometimes subliminal—about what is acceptable to feel, to say, or to desire. Perhaps a parent once admonished curiosity about one's own body, or a religious authority framed sexual thoughts as sinful. These early experiences lodge in the psyche as rules and prohibitions that persist into adulthood. Inner-child work involves entering into a compassionate conversation with the younger version of yourself who first heard those rules. In a quiet, reflective moment—perhaps in a journal or a guided meditation—you imagine yourself at that pivotal age, sitting beside your child-self. You speak gently: "I know you were told that your body is dirty, that feeling pleasure is bad. I'm sorry you carried that message." You listen as the child offers her fears: "I thought I was wrong to ask questions." You respond with reassurance: "It's safe now. You can ask, you can explore, and you can love your body unconditionally."

These dialogues may take the form of letters read aloud, conversations held in the mirror, or written scripts exchanged between your present self and your inner child. Over successive sessions, the voice of internalized taboo softens, replaced by a consistent refrain of safety, curiosity, and acceptance. The child's raw emotions—shame, fear, confusion—can be acknowledged and held, while the adult self imparts wisdom and protection. In this way, the very roots of shame, planted in early experience, are gently unearthed and replanted in soil enriched by compassion.

Constructive self-compassion practices dovetail with shame resilience and inner-child work to replace self-judgment with self-inquiry. Many of us habitually berate ourselves for perceived sexual "failures"—moments when desire wanes, when communication falters, or when experiments disappoint. In those moments, instead of piling on criticism, we can ask ourselves: "What am I feeling right now? What does my body need?" For instance, if nervousness arises before an intimate conversation, a self-compassionate approach might begin with naming: "I feel anxious." Then, acknowledging the shared human condition, one might say: "Anxiety is a normal response to vulnerability. Others feel it, too." Finally, allowing that anxious part space and care, one might offer a small kindness: "May I give myself permission to speak slowly and ask for a pause if I feel overwhelmed."

Exercises in self-compassion often involve brief pauses throughout the day—moments in which you place a hand over your heart and breathe into the sensation, repeating a phrase such as "I am worthy of care" or "May I be kind to myself." These micro-practices create a reservoir of kindness that you can draw upon when shame threatens to hijack your confidence. Over time, the brain learns to associate self-compassionate touch and kindness with regulatory safety, reducing the intensity and duration of shame reactions.

Together, the strategies of naming-witnessing-reaching out, inner-child dialogues, and constructive self-compassion form an integrated toolkit for dismantling the architecture of shame and guilt. Naming transforms shame from an amorphous force into a discernible experience; witnessing allows it to be held without judgment; reaching out fractures its isolation; inner-child dialogues heal its origins; and self-compassion rewrites the ongoing narrative with curiosity and care. As women practice these techniques, they not only reclaim their right to desire but also cultivate the emotional freedom to speak their truths, to explore their bodies, and to enter relationships from a place of integrity rather than self-reproach.

In practical terms, integrating these practices into daily life can begin with small, intentional rituals. Perhaps each morning you dedicate five minutes to journaling about any recurring guilt or shame themes, naming them explicitly as shame, witnessing them through free-form reflection, and then formulating one sentence you might share with a safe confidante. In the afternoon, you might pause to place a hand on your heart and conduct a brief inner-child check-in: "What story am I carrying from my past that needs soothing?" Before sleep, you might recite a self-compassion mantra, allowing the kindness to sink into the body's night-time rest.

Over weeks and months, these seemingly modest actions accumulate into a profound shift: shame no longer lurks in the shadows, but is greeted with openness; inner child wounds are met with healing presence; self-judgment gives way to curiosity. In its place grows a sturdy sense of agency—an unshakeable conviction that your desires, boundaries, and experiences are your own to define. This reclamation of self is the heart of sexual empowerment, a foundation upon which all further exploration, connection, and liberation can flourish. In the chapters that follow, you will harness this newfound agency to build confidence, advocate for your needs, and participate fully in the ever-unfolding adventure of authentic intimacy.

9.2 Building Confidence through Practice

Gaining confidence in one's sexual life often follows the principle familiar to athletes and artists: mastery emerges through deliberate, consistent practice. For many women, solitude provides the ideal laboratory for this skill-building. A structured regimen of solo exploration might begin with carving out regular time—perhaps fifteen to twenty minutes twice a week—dedicated solely to tuning in to bodily sensations without expectation or judgment. At first, the practice may consist of simple breath-and-touch routines, using gentle pressure or caressing strokes to discover which rhythms and areas evoke comfort or arousal. A calendar or journal becomes an essential companion: after each session, noting what felt enlivening, what felt neutral, and what stirred curiosity transforms vague impressions into concrete data. Week by week, the schedule can introduce incremental variations—a new technique borrowed from a trusted resource, a shift in pace, a different position—so that over a month the practitioner builds a personalized repertoire. As confidence grows in solo contexts, so too does the ease of sharing discoveries with a partner, since the foundational knowledge of one's own body reduces anxiety and amplifies the pleasure of mutual exploration.

Outside of solitary practice, workshops led by reputable educators offer accelerated learning opportunities. Whether one's interest lies in tantric breathing techniques, the gentle art of erotic massage, or advanced breathwork designed to channel arousal, the quality of instruction matters deeply. Before enrolling, it pays to research instructors' credentials: look for those who carry relevant certifications, have established relationships with professional organizations, or who receive consistently positive testimonials from past participants. A reputable tantra instructor, for example, will emphasize consent, clear communication, and emotional safety as much as the physical postures or breathing patterns. An erotic massage workshop offered by a licensed massage therapist will include anatomical lessons about nerve clusters and attention to potential contraindications. And a breathwork facilitator with training in trauma-informed approaches will guide participants through exercises that elevate heart rate and sensation without overwhelming the nervous system. Choosing workshops with transparent agendas, clear refund policies, and opportunities to ask questions in advance helps ensure that the learning environment remains respectful, evidence-based, and supportive of each woman's agency.

Yet no amount of external instruction replaces the power of feedback loops—ongoing cycles of action, reflection, and adjustment that refine preferences and strengthen confidence. After a solo session, one might review journal notes and extract a few insights: perhaps that a certain stroke pattern along the inner thigh elicited unexpected warmth, or that a particular breathing cadence created a sense of grounding rather than arousal. Translating these revelations into partner work involves sharing observations in simple, positive language: "Last night I noticed that slow, circular motions here felt really soothing—would you explore that with me?" Encouraging partners to reciprocate—by asking for feedback on their touch or pace—creates a collaborative laboratory in which both people learn to attune to each other's bodies. These dialogues need not be formal or clinical; they can arise naturally in the moment, or during a relaxed conversation over tea. The key is to reinforce that preferences are neither fixed nor shameful, but living data points subject to revision and growth.

Over months, the combined effect of solo regimens, quality workshops, and thoughtful feedback loops yields transformative results. Women report a growing sense of competence—no longer waiting for external validation to feel worthy of pleasure, but trusting their ability to direct their own experience. Partners, in turn, become more confident and responsive when they see that clear communication about likes and dislikes enhances intimacy rather than detracting from its spontaneity. Perhaps most importantly, the practice of building confidence through incremental mastery spills over into other areas of life: greater ease in setting boundaries at work, clearer articulation of needs in friendships, and a stronger sense of autonomy in pursuing personal goals. In this way, the lessons of sexual agency become a template for wholehearted living, where every act of self-discovery renews the promise of mutual respect, vulnerability, and joy.

9.3 Advocacy, Community & Collective Action

Sexual empowerment does not stop at the threshold of individual transformation; it flourishes most richly when women join together to build communities and champion broader cultural change. Grassroots campaigns offer a powerful mechanism for translating personal agency into collective breakthroughs. Imagine forming a small alliance of local women—friends, neighbors, or colleagues—with a shared vision of normalizing sex-positive education in the community. The first step might involve hosting a free workshop in a community center or library, where facilitators guide participants through foundational concepts such as consent, pleasure mapping, and boundary-setting. A simple template for launching such an event could include drafting a clear mission statement ("To provide inclusive, inclusive, non-judgmental sexual education for all adults"), securing a venue with flexible seating and privacy options, and recruiting speakers or panelists whose perspectives span diverse identities and experiences. Flyers distributed in local cafés, social media posts targeted to neighborhood groups, and partnerships with health clinics or bookstores amplify reach. As participants gather, the workshop not only imparts valuable information but also nurtures a sense of solidarity—women realize they are not alone in their questions, curiosities, and concerns.

Beyond in-person gatherings, digital activism has emerged as an essential front in reshaping narratives around female sexuality. Social media platforms—when used strategically—can amplify voices and normalize a wide array of expressions. A well-crafted campaign might begin with a hashtag that encapsulates a core message, such as #OwnYourPleasure or #BodiesInBloom. Individuals share short testimonials, artwork, or micro-blogs that speak to their own journeys: the relief of discovering menopause as a time of renewal, the courage of negotiating consent in a new relationship, or the pride of building confidence through a dance workshop. Influencers and grassroots organizers collaborate to post consistent content—interviews with experts, book recommendations, myth-busting infographics—ensuring that algorithms favor the material through regular engagement. Crucially, digital activism must maintain a commitment to privacy and consent: individuals sharing personal narratives do so at their own pace, with the option to remain anonymous or to use pseudonyms. By saturating online spaces with authentic, affirming messages, digital activists help dismantle the stigmas that have long silenced women's voices.

Sustained change, however, thrives not only through campaigns but also through intentional mentorship and allyship—intergenerational networks that knit together experience and innovation. A mentorship program might pair young women in their twenties or thirties with elders who have navigated decades of cultural shifts, providing guidance on everything from reproductive choices to the stewardship of relationship patterns. These relationships can take many forms: formal monthly check-ins, informal coffee meetups, or ongoing correspondence via email or messaging apps. The mentor offers historical context—how conversations about women's pleasure have evolved over time—while the mentee shares fresh insights on emerging technologies or contemporary cultural currents. Both parties learn and grow, forging bonds that transcend age-related divides and cultivate a continuum of sexual knowledge.

Allies, too, hold an essential place in this ecosystem. Men and nonbinary individuals who commit to supporting women's empowerment act as catalysts for broader cultural acceptance. They attend women-led workshops, amplify women's voices in mixed-gender forums, and model respectful communication in their own relationships. By scaffolding women's leadership rather than speaking over it, allies help ensure that sex-positive advocacy remains rooted in those most affected by its stigmas. In practical terms, an ally might volunteer at local events, sponsor workshop venues, or leverage workplace influence to secure inclusive health benefits that cover sexual health services. These collaborative efforts reinforce the idea that sexual empowerment is not an isolated struggle but a shared opportunity to enrich the well-being of entire communities.

As grassroots campaigns sow awareness at the local level, digital activism scales messages to global audiences, and mentorship weaves intergenerational wisdom into personal growth, the resulting tapestry of advocacy transcends any single initiative. What emerges is a culture in which open conversations about pleasure, consent, and agency become as routine as discussions about nutrition or cardiovascular health. In such a culture, women do not merely survive the legacies of shame and silencing; they thrive as authors of their own narratives, emboldened by the power of community, the reach of technology, and the solidarity of mentors and allies. This collective momentum lays the groundwork for lasting social change—one that honors diversity of experience, celebrates authentic expression, and affirms that every woman has the right to claim her sexual agency and pursue the intimacy she both desires and deserves.

Chapter 10: Authentic Expression & Creative Rituals

10.1 Erotic Art, Journaling & Creative Play

Ritual and creativity in sexuality spark the brain's reward centers more deeply than routine alone, inviting fresh neural pathways and amplifying the sense of novelty that underlies profound pleasure. In this final chapter, we turn our attention to the playful, imaginative side of intimacy—where art, words, and shared projects become conduits for authentic expression, deeper connection, and transformative insight. Through guided erotic sketching, stream-of-consciousness journaling, and dyadic creative collaborations, you will learn to infuse your sexual life with the spontaneity and wonder that often lie at the heart of the most unforgettable experiences.

The practice of sketching erotic art may feel intimidating at first—many women hold persistent beliefs that they are "not artistic" or that drawing bodies engages shame rather than celebration. Yet the goal here is not technical mastery but the tactile exploration of form, color, and emotion. To begin, gather a small sketchbook, a selection of colored pencils or charcoal sticks, and a private, comfortable space where you can focus without interruption. Your first prompt might be as simple as "draw a curve that feels like pleasure." Without lifting the pencil, let your hand trace a line across the page that reflects your internal sense of a wave, an arch, a swoop—whatever comes to mind when you remember a moment of sensation. Notice how the line accelerates or slows, where it widens or tapers, and allow those qualities to inform the shape.

After a few warm-up pages, introduce an image or memory as inspiration. You might recall the feeling of a late-summer breeze brushing against bare skin, or the warmth of a partner's hand on the small of your back. Sketch an abstract representation of that moment, using color to evoke temperature—cool blues for a light touch, warm reds or oranges for a firmer embrace. As you sketch, pay attention to the emotional undercurrents: does a jagged line feel more truthful than a smooth arc? Does a sudden shift in hue bring to mind surprise or delight? Resist any urge to judge your artistic choices; this is an exercise in embodied storytelling, not a performance for an external audience. Each stroke records an aspect of your sensory experience and lays the groundwork for deeper understanding.

Over successive sessions, your sketchbook becomes a visual diary of erotic discovery. You may notice recurring motifs—a spiral that signals rising desire, a cluster of small circles that suggests multiple points of sensitivity, a jagged edge that reflects a moment of tension or hesitation. By honoring these forms, you cultivate a more nuanced vocabulary for your own pleasure, one that cannot easily be captured in words alone. If you share your sketches with a trusted partner, the images can serve as conversation starters: "When I drew this looping shape in red, I was thinking of the warmth of your fingertips. Can we explore that sensation again?" In this way, erotic art bridges the private and the interpersonal, translating subjective experience into a shared language of color and contour.

Complementing visual exploration, daily stream-of-consciousness journaling unlocks subconscious themes that shape your intimate world. Set aside ten minutes at a consistent time each day—perhaps first thing in the morning or just before bed—and begin by writing a single prompt at the top of the page:

"Today I feel desire when..." or "My body remembers..." Then, without pausing to edit or censor, write continuously. Let your pen move freely, capturing every fleeting thought, memory, or association that arises. You might begin by noting a dream fragment, then segue into a recollection of a time when a partner's voice felt especially enticing, and then land on a question: "What would it feel like to reclaim that sense of anticipation now?"

Resist the temptation to impose structure or critique the flow—this raw material is precisely what reveals the patterns and narratives you may have overlooked. Over weeks, themes begin to surface: perhaps a particular song resurfaces, tied to a potent memory; or you discover an undercurrent of reverence for your own body's shape and texture. When the ten-minute timer chimes, read over what you have written and circle or underline passages that resonate most strongly. These marked lines become seeds for further exploration—perhaps a journaling session devoted to unpacking that one moment in greater depth, or a sketch that seeks to render the felt quality of that phrase in color and form.

Journaling and sketching feed into one another, forming a creative ecosystem that brings buried perspectives to light. If a journal entry repeatedly drifts toward a sense of longing for connection, a sketch might give that longing a visual counterpart—a pair of arcs nearly touching, a shape suspended in space. Conversely, a swirl drawn one afternoon may prompt a written reflection on the circumstances in which you first encountered that pattern. Over time, you build an integrated archive of self-generated prompts and responses, each layer adding texture to your evolving pleasure map.

To expand beyond solitary creativity, dyadic projects invite partners into the process of co-creation, forging new dimensions of intimacy. One accessible approach is to craft a joint vision board: together, you gather magazines, printed images, fabric swatches, and small found objects that symbolize the kinds of connection and pleasure you both wish to cultivate. On a large poster board or cork panel, arrange these elements in a collage— perhaps placing a photograph of intertwined hands near the center to represent mutual support, or a swatch of silk at the edge to symbolize tactile exploration. As you work side by side, conversation naturally flows: memories are shared, desires articulated, boundaries clarified. The vision board becomes a living artifact of your shared intention, one that can be revisited and updated in the months ahead.

Another dyadic option involves story-making: take turns contributing lines to a romantic or sensual narrative. One partner might begin, "She walked into the room and noticed the soft glow of candlelight dancing across the walls," and the other continues, "Her heart fluttered as she realized this space was a gift just for her." Building a collaborative story in this way encourages both partners to inhabit creative roles—author, listener, editor—and to practice turning ideas into evocative language. The story need not culminate in explicit sexual detail; its power lies in the shared imagination of atmosphere, emotion, and anticipation. Once written, you might read the narrative aloud to each other in a quiet evening gathering, laying the words as soft music beneath a ritual of gentle touch or synchronized breath.

Engaging in these creative rituals transforms intimacy into a co-crafted phenomenon rather than an act of consumption. Each sketch, journal entry, or collage piece becomes a testament to vulnerability and curiosity, reinforcing the message that your desires are not quirks to be hidden but seeds to be nurtured. As the habit of creative play takes root, you may find that unexpected insights emerge—perhaps a buried fantasy resurfaces in your freewrites, or a color palette in your sketches reveals a previously unarticulated preference for warmth and softness. These discoveries can guide future experiments in communication, bodywork, or sexual settings, ensuring that your practice remains responsive to the living currents of your inner world.

In building such a creative practice, it is essential to honor both spontaneity and ritual. While the initial act of free sketching or journaling thrives on unstructured exploration, integrating these practices into your weekly routine—setting aside specific times, creating a dedicated space, lighting a candle or playing soft music—confers a ritual quality that signals to the subconscious mind: "Now we step into the realm of imagination." Over time, the familiarity of the ritual amplifies its power, much like a meditation cushion or yoga mat cues the body to shift into reflective mode. Whether alone or with a partner, these creative rituals become anchors of self-discovery, reminding you that sexuality is as much an art as it is a physical act—an ever-unfolding canvas upon which you paint your most authentic expression.

By weaving together erotic art, journaling, and dyadic creative play, you cultivate a rich landscape of symbols, stories, and shapes that illuminate the deepest contours of your desire. In this space of playful experimentation, shame and routine lose their grip, replaced by a fluid dialogue between mind, body, and heart. As your sketches grow bolder, your journal pages more candid, and your collaborative projects more resonant, you step fully into the role of author and architect of your own sexual narrative—an empowered artist crafting, day by day, a masterpiece of authentic expression and enduring connection.

10.2 Designing Personal Rituals & Ceremonies

Rituals have shaped human culture for millennia, offering a structured way to mark passages of time, honor transitions, and anchor the unpredictable rhythms of life in moments of sacred intention. When applied to one's sexual wellbeing, personal rituals and ceremonies serve a similar function: they transform ordinary routines into meaningful acts of self-acknowledgment, deepen the mind–body connection, and open the heart to authentic expression. Three domains—moon-cycle celebrations, bedroom sanctification, and transition ceremonies—provide fertile ground for crafting practices that resonate with your own values and experiences.

Beginning with moon-cycle celebrations, one harnesses the ancient correspondence between the lunar phases and the menstrual cycle. Just as the moon waxes toward fullness and then wanes, our bodies move through phases of energy and rest: menstruation, the follicular growth phase, ovulation, and the luteal phase before the next bleed. A ritual for the menstrual phase might begin on the first day of bleeding, when many women feel called to inward reflection. A quiet ceremony could include lighting a single red or black candle, placing a small bowl of warm herbal tea (such as red raspberry leaf) on a windowsill, and reciting an affirmation like, "In this time of release, I honor the power of renewal." Some women choose to wear a specific piece of jewelry only during menstruation—a hematite ring or a garnet pendant—as a tactile reminder of their connection to the earth's cycles.

As the body shifts into the follicular phase, energy typically returns and creativity blossoms. A corresponding new-moon ritual might involve planting a seed—literal or metaphorical—in fertile soil or in a journal: writing down intentions for new projects, relationship goals, or explorations of pleasure you wish to cultivate in the coming weeks. You might include symbols of growth—a green candle, a small potted herb, or a hand-drawn spiral—placing them on a dedicated altar or tray that remains in view until ovulation. Speaking your intentions aloud, with unwavering confidence, enlists the mind's creative power and invites the universe to conspire in your favor.

When ovulation arrives, the body's energy peaks, often accompanied by heightened libido and a sense of expansiveness. A full-moon celebration can channel this vitality into a feast of gratitude and connection. Perhaps you invite a close friend or partner to share a ceremony of abundance: arranging a platter of fresh fruit, dark chocolate, and herbal elixirs, lighting silver or white candles, and taking turns speaking aloud what you most appreciate about your bodies and desires. The fullness of the moon's light mirrors the fullness of your own capacity for pleasure and connection, reminding you that abundance is not only possible but deserved.

In the luteal phase, as the moon wanes and energy begins to ebb, a ceremony of letting go can ease the transition into rest. You might write down lingering stressors—unfinished work tasks, emotional burdens, interpersonal tensions—on small strips of biodegradable paper. In a safe outdoor space or over a candle, you burn these slips, watching the smoke carry away what no longer serves you. A closing blessing—spoken softly or sung—marks your readiness to surrender and retreat into the next cycle's inward phase.

Across all these lunar-menstrual ceremonies, the consistent elements are intentionality, symbolism, and sensory engagement. The flicker of candlelight establishes a container of safety; the tactile act of planting seeds or burning paper anchors the mind in the body; spoken words give shape to the inner landscape. Over months and years, these rituals become more than occasional events—they form an ongoing dialogue with your cyclical nature, building respect for the wisdom encoded in your hormones and the lunar orbit alike.

In parallel with lunar-cycle rituals, bedroom sanctification transforms the space of intimacy into a sanctuary of presence. The bedroom often doubles as an office, a reading nook, or a spot for late-night scrolling, diluting its potential as a site of ritual. To reclaim it, begin by clearing clutter: tuck away work materials, organize fabrics, and designate one shelf or table as your "altar." On this altar, place objects that remind you of your values and intentions: a small vase of fresh flowers, a favorite crystal or stone, a framed affirmation card, or a dedicated journal.

Lighting is integral to atmosphere. Soft, layered illumination—combining dimmable lamps, strings of fairy lights, and unscented candles—encourages the parasympathetic relaxation necessary for intimacy. Avoid harsh overhead fixtures; instead, opt for warm-toned bulbs that mimic sunset's glow. A plug-in essential-oil diffuser can fill the air with scents associated with calm and openness—lavender to soothe, rose to evoke compassion, ylang-ylang to lift the spirit.

Soundscapes complete the sanctification. A curated playlist—perhaps instrumental tracks with gentle rhythms, nature recordings of ocean waves or rainforest birds, or low-frequency binaural beats designed to entrain the brain to a state of deep relaxation—guides the mind away from daily worries. Place a small Bluetooth speaker near the altar, and keep volume at a level that permits conversation as well as introspection.

To formally open the sanctified space, you might create a ritual each time you prepare for intimacy. Stand at the threshold of the bedroom, take three grounding breaths, and speak an invocation: "In this space, love and safety dwell. May my body and heart open here." Stepping inside, you pause to touch each object on your altar, acknowledging its significance. Only then do you lie down, engage with your partner, or move into solo practice—whatever form your intimacy takes. This act of mindful transition signals to the nervous system that the time for rest, play, or connection has begun, reducing the habitual mental clutter that often intrudes at night.

Ritual design extends most poignantly to transition ceremonies—those rites that mark significant shifts in life phase. After childbirth, for example, the body and identity undergo seismic transformation. A postpartum ceremony might center on the placenta, honoring it as sacred intermediary between mother and child. Wrapped in cloth and placed beneath a special plant in the garden, the placenta becomes the seed of new life, and the ritual of planting symbolizes the mother's own emergence into a transformed state. Following a gentle blessing—spoken by a supportive circle of friends or family—the new mother may perform a water ritual, soaking in a tub infused with healing herbs such as calendula and rose petals, while loved ones offer supportive touch or supportive words.

When perimenopause transitions into menopause, another kind of ceremony can honor the closing of one chapter and the opening of another. A symbolic act might involve writing a letter to your menstrual cycle—thanking it for the gifts of fertility, creative surges of energy, and deep self-knowledge—and then releasing the letter into running water or burning it in a small, contained fire bowl. As smoke or water carries away the words, you feel a sense of release from once-rigid expectations around periodic bleeding. To honor the arrival of a new phase, you might don a special scarf or piece of jewelry—perhaps amber or moonstone—that you will wear in subsequent months as a talisman of second blooming.

Across all transition rituals, the elements of symbolism, communal support, and sensory engagement coalesce to mark change not with anxiety but with celebration and acceptance. By crafting ceremonies that reflect the depth of each life passage—whether the emergence of motherhood, the shedding of a cycle, or any other rite of passage—you create meaningful bookends around transformations that might otherwise be met with confusion or loss. Instead, each transition becomes an invitation to claim agency, celebrate resilience, and step forward with intentional grace.

10.3 Technology, Virtual Intimacy & Future Trends

In an era when smartphones, virtual reality headsets, and artificial intelligence shape nearly every aspect of daily life, technology's role in sexuality is rapidly expanding. What was once confined to erotica now encompasses haptic devices that simulate touch across distances, VR platforms that transport users to immersive intimate environments, and AI-driven apps that function as personalized intimacy coaches. Navigating these innovations demands both curiosity and caution, as the promise of expanded connection coexists with ethical complexities around data privacy, consent, and inclusivity.

Haptic and virtual reality platforms represent the cutting edge of remote intimacy. Haptic suits and gloves, equipped with an array of sensors and actuators, translate digital interactions into tactile feedback—gentle pulses, pressure changes, or simulated stroking patterns—on the recipient's body. Paired with VR headsets displaying rendered environments, users can inhabit shared spaces where avatars move and touch in real time, their gestures reflected in synchronized haptic sensations. Early adopters describe the thrill of a partner's virtual hand sliding along their forearm, the illusion heightened by 3D audio cues and the absence of external distractions. Beyond the novelty of simulated presence, these technologies hold promise for couples separated by distance, individuals exploring solo sensual experiences with guided programs, and communities seeking to normalize non-physical forms of intimacy for those with limited mobility.

Yet haptic-VR technologies are not without limitations. Latency between movement and sensation can disrupt the illusion, leaving users disoriented rather than immersed. The fidelity of touch—its warmth, texture, and subtle modulation—remains a challenge for engineers, as current devices approximate rather than replicate the nuanced feedback of human skin. Moreover, cost and accessibility pose barriers: high-end haptic suits run into the thousands of dollars, and VR headsets require powerful computers or consoles. As a result, early adopters often skew toward tech-savvy demographics, risking the reinforcement of inequalities in sexual access and innovation.

Parallel to haptic-VR, artificial intelligence is carving a niche as an intimacy coach—a digital companion that offers personalized guidance based on user input and behavioral data. Emerging apps invite users to log moods, track partner feedback, and note patterns of desire or avoidance. The AI then analyzes these data points, drawing on large language models and behavioral algorithms to suggest tailored exercises: a breathwork sequence for evening relaxation, a communication script for negotiating consent, or a gentle reminder to schedule partner check-ins. Some platforms integrate biofeedback from wearable devices—heart rate variability, skin temperature, or sleep quality—refining their recommendations in near-real time. Beta-testers report that the unobtrusive, judgment-free presence of an AI coach reduces anxiety around performance and provides accountability in sustaining new habits.

However, the integration of AI into intimate realms raises pressing ethical considerations. First and foremost is digital consent: users must understand what data are collected, how they are stored, and who can access them. Unlike fitness trackers, which capture step counts and heart rates, intimacy coaches record deeply personal reflections on desire, boundaries, and relationship dynamics. Without robust encryption and transparent privacy policies, this information could be exploited for targeted marketing, non-consensual surveillance, or malicious uses. Ethical frameworks emphasize that data ownership should remain firmly with the user, that explicit, revocable consent is required for each category of data, and that any sharing with third parties must be opt-in rather than opt-out.

Inclusivity represents another challenge. AI models trained on narrow datasets risk reinforcing stereotypes or excluding marginalized identities. An intimacy coach that interprets patterns solely through a heterosexual, cisnormative lens may misread the experiences of LGBTQ+ users or those with non-traditional relationship structures. To guard against such biases, developers must collaborate with diverse communities in the design, testing, and iterating of AI algorithms, ensuring that prompts, recommendations, and user interfaces reflect a broad spectrum of lived experiences.

Looking ahead, the convergence of haptics, VR, and AI suggests a future of hybrid intimacy—where physical and virtual worlds blend seamlessly. Augmented reality (AR) glasses might project a partner's avatar into one's living room, complete with spatial audio and touch feedback. Blockchain technologies could secure micro-transactions for sharing personal erotic art or guided meditations, empowering creators with direct compensation models. Neural interfaces, while still in early experimental stages, could eventually translate thought-initiated commands into haptic or visual stimuli, bypassing manual controls altogether. Each innovation carries the potential to enrich connection, creativity, and sexual exploration—but only if guided by ethical guardrails that prioritize consent, privacy, and equity.

As we stand at the threshold of these emerging landscapes, the question is not whether technology will transform intimacy—it already has—but how we choose to shape that transformation. By engaging critically with haptic devices, VR platforms, AI coaches, and the ethical frameworks that govern them, women and their allies can ensure that the future of virtual intimacy remains rooted in respect for autonomy, celebration of diversity, and unwavering commitment to shared pleasure and wellbeing. In this way, technology becomes not a substitute for genuine human connection, but an amplifier of the infinite possibilities that arise when creativity, consent, and compassion intersect.

Conclusions

"Sexual wellbeing is not a destination but an ever-evolving journey of self-discovery and connection."

As we draw this handbook to a close, it is worth pausing to honor the incredible terrain we have traversed together. From the neural circuitry that underpins arousal to the somatic practices that attune us to the body's whispers, from the pleasure mapping that reveals our unique sensual blueprints to the communication models that transform consent into an act of love, every chapter has offered a piece of the mosaic that constitutes holistic sexual health. We began by recognizing that the brain is our most powerful sexual organ and moved outward through layers of embodiment, emotional intimacy, and creative expression. By integrating ancient wisdom traditions alongside cutting-edge science, this guide has shown that physical sensation, emotional safety, social connection, and spiritual meaning are not separate spheres but threads woven into a single tapestry.

In revisiting the journey's milestones, we see how each domain reinforced and enriched the others. The neurobiology of pleasure taught us why anticipation and attachment matter, illuminating the roles of dopamine, oxytocin, and endorphins in shaping our experience of desire. Those insights seamlessly informed our somatic awareness work—body scans, mindful touch, and progressive muscle relaxation—by revealing the importance of tuning our nervous systems toward safety and receptivity. With that foundation in place, we charted personalized pleasure maps, documenting sensations, contexts, and emotional states until we could navigate our own bodies with the confidence of an explorer mapping familiar terrain.

Communication and consent emerged next as the scaffolding that supports every act of intimacy. Learning to use the simple yet powerful Yes/No/Maybe framework, to decode the subtleties of body language, and to craft safe words and signals taught us that clarity is an act of care. Building on these essentials, we embraced advanced communication tools—Nonviolent Communication templates and journal-based role-play—to express needs and boundaries with both honesty and empathy. At the same time, we discovered how digital platforms and physiological tracking devices could augment our dialogue, ensuring that consent and mutual understanding remain active components of our evolving relationships.

Our exploration of emotional intimacy led us through the landscape of attachment styles and provided the tools to shift toward secure attachment patterns, rituals that foster deep vulnerability, and healing modalities for past trauma. We celebrated the body's inherent wisdom, deconstructing harmful beauty myths through media literacy and cultivating body positivity with mirror work, dance improvisation, and art therapy. Hormonal health guided us from the first blush of puberty through the cycles of adulthood into the second blooming of menopause, equipping us with the language to understand our ever-shifting desires.

Holistic practices for sexual wellbeing wove together movement, breath, nutrition, and self-care. Yoga and dance awakened the pelvic floor and hip mobility; Pilates fortified the core; breathwork and meditation regulated the nervous system; adaptogens, micronutrients, and anti-inflammatory meals nurtured our biochemistry. Integrating sexuality with overall wellness, we recognized the importance of strength, endurance, and flexibility, of restful sleep and strategic napping, and of mental health supports that combine therapy, coaching, and community.

Next, in our study of empowerment and agency, we confronted shame and guilt—those silent thieves of desire—armed with shame-resilience practices, inner-child dialogues, and self-compassion. We learned to build confidence through structured solo exploration, skill-building workshops, and feedback loops that refine our preferences. We amplified our impact by embracing advocacy, from grassroots workshops to digital activism and intergenerational mentorship, weaving our personal insights into the broader fabric of social change.

Finally, in this culminating chapter on authentic expression and creative rituals, we tapped into the transformative power of erotic art, stream-of-consciousness journaling, and dyadic vision-boarding. We sanctified intimate spaces with rites that honor the menstrual cycle, purify our bedrooms, and celebrate life's transitions. And we looked ahead, exploring the frontiers of virtual intimacy—haptic devices, VR platforms, AI coaches—while insisting on ethical frameworks that safeguard consent, privacy, and inclusion.

If each chapter has contributed a vital strand to this tapestry, the thread that binds them all is your own embodied agency. This handbook offers maps and tools, research and rituals, but the journey itself is yours to chart. To carry forward everything you have learned, consider designing a personalized "Sexual Wellbeing Plan." Begin by reflecting on the areas where you feel most grounded—perhaps you have already mastered coherent breathing or have built a robust pleasure map—and those where you sense potential for growth—maybe your inner-child dialogues still feel tentative, or you have yet to explore nutrition strategies for hormonal balance. In a dedicated journal or digital document, write down three to five intentions that integrate practices from different chapters: a commitment to daily coherent breathing during your luteal phase, weekly mirror work complemented by monthly creative collaborations with a partner, quarterly reviews of your digital consent tools, or the launch of a small community workshop on body positivity.

Each intention should be paired with concrete actions and milestones. If you wish to deepen your somatic awareness, schedule ten-minute body scans every morning for two weeks, then evaluate whether you can sustain that practice or whether adjustments—perhaps a different time of day or an alternative posture—would work better. If you aim to strengthen your pelvic floor, outline a progression of Kegel holds and pulses, noting when to introduce resistance bands or biofeedback devices. Should you aspire to creative expression, earmark specific blocks of time for sketching, journaling, or vision boarding, and identify accountability partners who will join you or celebrate your progress. By weaving together pieces from multiple chapters into a coherent plan, you ensure that your approach remains balanced, dynamic, and aligned with your deepest values.

Maintaining momentum requires ongoing support and continued growth. Consider curating a personal library of resources: key books on neurobiology, communication, and somatic therapies; bookmarked online articles on cycle charting and hormone health; links to reputable podcasts and YouTube channels on sexual empowerment. Join peer communities—whether in-person groups, coaching pods, or moderated online forums—where you can share insights, troubleshoot challenges, and bask in the resonance of shared experience. Seek out professional support when needed: a sex-positive therapist to navigate complex emotions, a pelvic floor physiotherapist to guide you through advanced myofascial release, a certified breathwork facilitator to refine your coherence practices.

In this spirit of lifelong learning, remember that the path of sexual wellbeing is rarely linear. Life circumstances evolve—new relationships emerge, stress levels fluctuate, health conditions arise, technology advances—and each shift invites a recalibration of our practices and intentions. What felt nourishing in one season may require adaptation in the next. Yet with the holistic framework you now possess—grounded in science, rooted in wisdom traditions, and enlivened by creative play—you are uniquely equipped to meet each transition with curiosity, resilience, and compassion.

May this handbook serve not only as a reference guide but as a trusted companion on your ongoing voyage of self-discovery. May its pages remind you that pleasure, consent, embodiment, and authenticity are not luxury pursuits but essential facets of human flourishing. Above all, may you carry forward the understanding that sexual wellbeing is not a box to be checked but a living, breathing journey—one that invites you, every day, to connect more deeply with yourself, with others, and with the inexhaustible wellspring of life itself.

www.ingramcontent.com/pod-product-compliance
Lightning Source LLC
Chambersburg PA
CBHW062035200326
41519CB00017B/5043